Mental Health and Personalisation

Themes and issues in recovery-based mental health care and support

Daisy Bogg

Social Perspectives Network
for modern mental health

Pavilion

Mental Health and Personalisation

Themes and issues in recovery-based mental health care and support

Published by:
Pavilion Publishing (Brighton) Ltd
Richmond House
Richmond Road
Brighton
BN2 3RL

Tel: 01273 623222
Fax: 01273 625526
Email: info@pavpub.com
Web: www.pavpub.com

First published 2010

A catalogue record for this book is available from the British Library.

ISBN: 978-1-84196-280-1

Pavilion is the leading training and development provider and publisher in the health, social care and allied fields, providing a range of innovative training solutions underpinned by sound research and professional values. We aim to put our customers first, through excellent customer service and value.

Author: Daisy Bogg, on behalf of SPN
Editor: Kerry Boettcher, Pavilion
Cover design: Anthony Pitt, Pavilion
Page layout and typesetting: Emma Garbutt, Pavilion
Printing: Ashford Press

Contents

Acknowledgements

Thanks are due to SPN who have supported and promoted this workbook and co-ordinated much of the process.

Thanks are due to the Department of Health for financial support for this publication.

This has been a very collaborative project and thanks are due to everyone who has been involved. My thanks to the steering group for their feedback and comments on each section, it has been helpful to have different views and interpretations of what each capability is about.

As always, thanks are due to my family and friends, most notably my husband Terry who made me lots of cups of tea and didn't moan too much about being neglected by my work.

About the author

Daisy Bogg is an executive committee member of the Social Perspectives Network (SPN) and executive director of Social Care and Specialist Services for Bedfordshire and Luton Partnership NHS Trust. Daisy is a social worker by background and has worked within mental health and addiction services for the last 15 years. She has written postgraduate texts on the integration of social work into the NHS and the values and ethics of mental health practice. She also writes a regular column in Mental Health Today magazine on behalf of SPN. Daisy is now in independent practice, running a training and consultancy company and is available to facilitate training and development.

About the Social Perspectives Network

The Social Perspectives Network is a coalition of service users, carers, policy makers, academics and practitioners who are interested in how social factors contribute to people becoming distressed, and play a crucial part in promoting recovery. The SPN aims to share work and information on mental health from a social perspective, to support people to put social perspectives into practice, and influence the development of mental health policy.

Steering group

The steering group for this publication was made up of professionals, policy makers, academics, service users and carers, all of whom have provided invaluable insights and feedback throughout the process of compiling this workbook.

Robin Murray-Neill, Department of Health, Putting People First (Delivery) Team

Sarah Carr, Senior Research Analyst, Social Care Institute for Excellence

Raza Griffiths, Joint Project Co-ordinator, SPN

Alleyn Wilson, Co-chair, SPN; Chair of Trustees, SPN and Carer

Jenny Robb, Deputy Director of Social Care, Mersey Care NHS Trust

Tina Coldham, National Development Consultant, HASCAS

Terry Bamford, Trustee, SPN

Dr Ruth Allen, Director of Social Work, South West London and St George's Mental Health NHS Trust

Jane Banning, SDS Support Lead, Cambridgeshire County Council

Julie Lunt, Mental Health Lead, Helen Sanderson Associates

Introduction

Personalisation in mental health services is a subject that encompasses many areas and meanings, from social inclusion principles through to a simple direct payment, and as such, this workbook aims to assist service users, carers and professionals to work through the themes and issues as related to recovery-based mental health care and support.

The Putting People First concordant, which was published in 2007 (LGA, ADASS, NHS, 2007), was the first cross-governmental agreement that was developed to capture the universal nature of the transformation process and the government's commitment to making this vision a reality. Subsequent work, by the Putting People First (PPF) project team, has further developed this vision and identified the four key areas of personalisation:

- universal services
- early intervention and prevention
- choice and control
- social capital

Choice and control form the basis of the approach, with increased service user control and the application of person-centred approaches, as well as initiatives such as direct payments and personal budgets, which are designed to enable individual control over support packages. Universal services emphasise the social inclusion aspects of support and encourage access to mainstream and community services as part of the support process. Social capital draws upon the wider social context, considering informal support and community involvement as key elements of an individual's well-being, and finally early intervention and prevention focus on overall well-being, public health issues and preventative services that address social and health issues and prevent individuals from experiencing mental health issues in the first instance as the preferred option.

This approach has also been supported by wider government agendas, with a new mental health policy New Horizons published in 2009, which stated personalisation was fundamental to recovery, and personalised approaches are also being introduced across health and social care as the preferred method of public sector support.

Mental health services and support have been an integrated health and social care approach for some time, which means that different approaches and professional perspectives need to be co-ordinated and combined. Work undertaken in the early 2000s attempted to establish a common set of competencies which all workers involved in delivering mental health support would need to develop and demonstrate. The 10 Essential Shared Capabilities was published in 2004 as the framework for all, and this workbook draws on these capabilities to demonstrate and explore how the personalisation agenda can be delivered in an integrated mental health setting.

The 10 Essential Shared Capabilities

This workbook is presented in 10 sections, which each relate to the Essential Shared Capabilities (Hope, 2004). Each section applies the capabilities to different aspects of personalisation and a range of activities are used to enable the reader to develop their understanding of both frameworks and consider the issues within their local context.

While this framework was originally created for the workforce, the nature of personalisation means that service users and carers are equal partners within the care and support processes, and as such, the commentary and activities included within this workbook are designed to be applicable across the whole range of stakeholders with an interest in mental health and mental health services.

The areas that will be considered throughout this workbook are as follows.

Section 1: Working in partnership

Developing and maintaining constructive working relationships with service users, carers, families, colleagues, lay people and wider community networks. Working positively with any tensions created by conflicts of interest or aspiration that may arise between the partners in care.

Section 2: Respecting diversity

Working in partnership with service users, carers, families and colleagues to provide care and interventions that not only make a positive difference but also do so in ways that respect and value diversity including age, race, culture, disability, gender, spirituality and sexuality.

Section 3: Practising ethically

Recognising the rights and aspirations of service users and their families, acknowledging power differentials and minimising them whenever possible. Providing treatment and care that is accountable to service users and carers within the boundaries prescribed by national (professional), legal and local codes of ethical practice.

Section 4: Challenging inequality

Addressing the causes and consequences of stigma, discrimination, social inequality and exclusion on service users, carers and mental health services. Creating, developing or maintaining valued social roles for people in the communities they come from.

Section 5: Promoting recovery

Working in partnership to provide care and treatment that enables service users and carers to tackle mental health problems with hope and optimism and to work towards a valued lifestyle within and beyond the limits of any mental health problem.

Section 6: Identifying people's needs and strengths

Working in partnership to gather information to agree health and social care needs in the context of the preferred lifestyle and aspirations of service users their families, carers and friends.

Section 7: Providing service user-centred care

Negotiating achievable and meaningful goals, primarily from the perspective of service users and their families. Influencing and seeking the means to achieve these goals and clarifying the responsibilities of the people who will provide any help that is needed, including systematically evaluating outcomes and achievements.

Section 8: Making a difference

Facilitating access to and delivering the best quality, evidence-based, values-based health and social care interventions to meet the needs and aspirations of service users and their families and carers.

Section 9: Promoting safety and positive risk taking

Empowering the person to decide the level of risk they are prepared to take with their health and safety. This includes working with the tension between promoting safety and positive risk taking, including assessing and dealing with possible risks for service users, carers, family members, and the wider public.

Section 10: Personal development and learning

Keeping up-to-date with changes in practice and participating in life-long learning, personal and professional development for one's self and colleagues through supervision, appraisal and reflective practice.

The capabilities are each divided into a set of competencies taken from the original guidance, and this workbook applies the themes, issues and principles of personalisation to each competence. The aim is to assist readers to work through a range of areas within the framework of competent mental health practice, and to develop their knowledge and skills in relation to delivering personalised mental health support.

References

Hope R (2004) *The 10 Essential Shared Capabilities: A framework for the whole of the mental health workforce*. London: DH.

LGA, ADASS, NHS (2007) *Putting People First: A shared vision and commitment to the transformation of adult social care*. London: DH.

Section 1: Working in partnership

Developing and maintaining constructive working relationships with service users, carers, families, colleagues, lay people and wider community networks. Working positively with any tensions created by conflicts of interest or aspirations that may arise between the partners in care.

This capability is concerned with the engagement of all those providing or receiving mental health services and support. Relationship building is a key skill for all those involved in the sector and is also a key theme within the personalisation of mental health care. There is significant evidence (Shattell, Starr & Thomas, 2007; McCabe & Priebe, 2004; Gilburt, Rose & Slade, 2008; Huxley *et al*, 2009) that the relationship between service user and care provider (whether formal or informal) has a significant impact upon the outcomes for all those involved, and personalisation reiterates this evidence by considering partnership between service user and provider as a core theme to the successful implementation.

Aims

The whole of this workbook is targeted at achieving the general aims as set out in the introductory section, however, each section also has specific aims, linked to the Essential Shared Capability it is exploring, as such, the aims of this section of the workbook are:

- to understand the range of definitions of personalisation in mental health and social care, and be able to articulate these meanings to build a shared understanding with service users, carers, communities and professionals
- to become aware of the benefits of working in partnership with the full range of stakeholders and how this can promote choice, control and citizenship
- to increase awareness of how partnership working can promote a recovery approach within responses to mental health difficulties.

Overview

Defining and articulating personalisation and what it means to service users and carers in real terms is the first focus of this workbook. There appears to be a wide range of interpretations of personalisation, and a common understanding of what is being worked towards is vital if partnership between stakeholders is to be achieved. As the reader works through this section, information and activities will be used to enable understanding and application to the local experience, with the aim being to assist in the development of a clear view of what personalisation means within the context of partnership working and to support competence within this area.

Six areas of competence are included within this first shared capability, these are:

Competence 1:	Have the ability to explain in an understandable way, their professional role and any parameters that they work within.
Competence 2:	Have the ability to communicate with all the stakeholders involved in an individual's care.
Competence 3:	Understand their role and that of others within a multidisciplinary setting.
Competence 4:	Be able to engage service users in a collaborative assessment process.
Competence 5:	Acknowledge the part that families and carers play in the service user's support network and be able to engage them as partners in care.
Competence 6:	Be able to communicate across disciplinary, professional and organisational boundaries.

By working through these competencies the reader will be able to identify the scope of the changes in both the national context and the local area, drawing on community resources and the whole system consideration of the 'mobilisation of services' to meet individual needs.

The activities within this section are aimed at assisting readers to scope-out the possible circle of support, how to communicate the range of options in plain English, and creating a local resource guide to promote the principle of 'information as a service'. Within these competency based exercises issues such as communication skills, co-production with service users and carers, social relationships, multidisciplinary working and engagement issues will be explored and each activity can be applied to a wide range of groups and experiences by drawing on local experiences within the context of personalisation and the recovery approach to mental health.

Competence 1

Developing the ability to explain, in an understandable way, their role and any parameters that they work within.

Personalisation is a term that is used extensively within mental health care, and the understanding and interpretation of its use is variable depending on the experience, perceptions and beliefs within which they are applied. These variations can cause difficulties for service users, carers and professionals as the lack of clarity has the potential to influence how individuals and groups work together, and how the ultimate goals of any support packages are understood. There are many definitions that can be found for the term personalisation, ranging from standard dictionary definitions through to more descriptive forms such as those presented here.

> *'...every person who receives support, whether provided by statutory services or funded by themselves, will be empowered to shape their own lives and the services they receive.'* (Office for Disability Issues, 2008)

> *'Personalisation means starting with the individual as a person with strengths and preferences who may have a network of support and resources, which can include family and friends.'* (Carr, 2008)

> *'...disabled people are "best placed" to take the lead in identifying their own needs and in identifying the most appropriate means of meeting them.'*
> (Hudson & Henwood, 2008)

> *'...the process by which state-provided services can be adapted to suit you. In social care this means everyone having choice and control over the shape of their support along with a greater emphasis on prevention and early interventions.'* (Finch, 2008)

> *'...dependent users become consumers and commissioners, and eventually co-producers and co-designers. Their participation, commitment, knowledge and responsibility increases. As the role of the user fills out, so the role of the professional must change in tandem.'* (Leadbetter, 2004)

There are a number of key themes that can be identified, the strongest of which appears to be that of service users taking control of the support they need and becoming partners in the process of assessment and care planning. The emphasis of personalisation to date, and certainly within the definitions presented, appears to be from a strong social care perspective, however, this is not the sole emphasis in the transformation process, and the full range of health, care, and community resources and facilities need to be considered within the personalisation debate.

For workers and service users to engage with personalisation, there is a need to develop the capability to articulate what is meant by the term, and to be able to present this in the context of the role they are playing within the process.

Activity: Defining personalisation – mind mapping

Creativity is a core component of personalisation, as it requires all stakeholders to think beyond traditional care methods and consider more widely what could be put in place to promote choice, control and independence for service users of mental health support services. Mind mapping can be used as a creative method of developing personal and communal definitions of personalised care. To be able to explain personalisation the individual first needs to understand what the term means and how this impacts upon their role – whether service user, carer or professional – this activity will assist the reader to define their own understanding.

Creating a mind map

This exercise can be carried out individually or in a group.

- Start in the centre of a sheet of blank paper – write the word 'personalisation' and add an image or drawing that you feel represents the term.
- Using branches (lines) leading from personalisation write down words that are linked to the term. Use single words or simple phrases for information. Most words in normal writing are padding, single strong words and meaningful phrases can convey the same meaning – excess words just clutter the mind map.
- Print words. Joined up or indistinct writing can be more difficult to read.
- Use colour to separate different ideas. This will help you to separate ideas and identify links.
- Use symbols and images. Where a symbol or picture means something to you, use it. Pictures can help you to remember information more effectively than words.

- Using cross-linkages. Information in one part of the mind map may relate to another part. Here you can draw in lines to show the cross-linkages. This helps you to see how one part of the subject connects with another.

Illustrated example

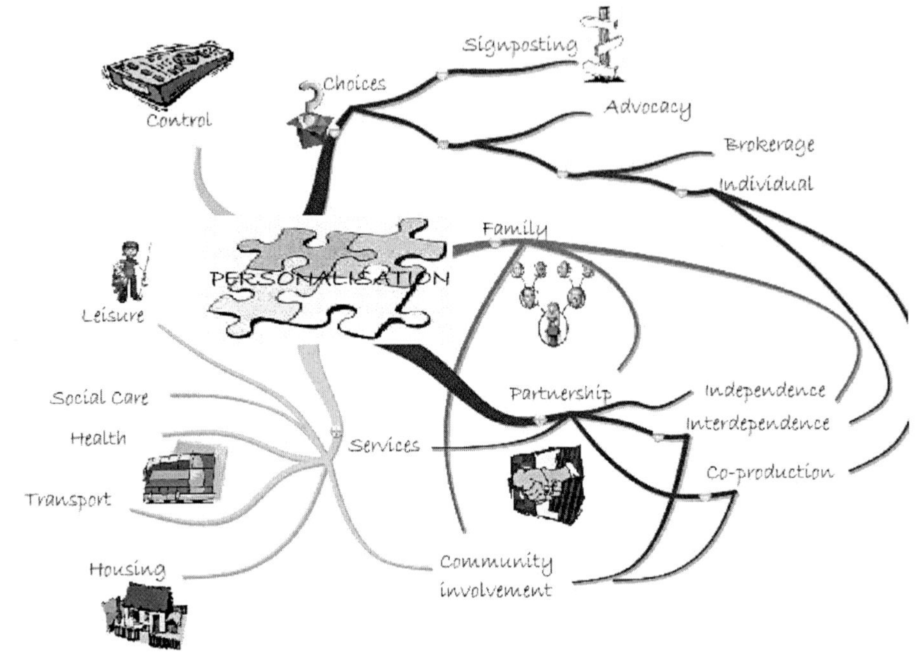

* Created using Buzan's iMindMap – available from http://www.mind-mapping.co.uk

This example is designed to assist in the process of thinking about how to start creating an individual mind map, and is provided for illustration purposes only. The concepts within the illustration should be developed into further branches to assist the conceptualisation of the terms and identify how they link together. A mind map is a dynamic process, and may be added to throughout the workbook to assist in defining and organising learning.

Once you have completed the initial mapping concerning the definitions and terms that make up a personalised approach, review your mind map and consider the following.

- What are the key themes of your approach?
- What is your definition of personalisation?
- What role do you play within this definition of personalisation?

Competence 2

Developing the ability to communicate with all the stakeholders involved in an individual's care.

Within a recovery context mental health support can be accessed from a wide range of sources, from family members and professional mental health teams, through to education providers, employers, community groups and social groups. As a result there is often a range of individuals involved in a service user's daily life that are not identified or acknowledged as part of the network in the assessment and care planning processes. The nature of personalised care supports the development of these types of diverse networks, as a means of promoting a personalised, more socially inclusive and normalised approach. As a result, those operating within the field will need to think outside the traditional 'box' and learn how to consider and communicate with a wider range of stakeholders.

The idea of social capital is a key theme in this competence, and as discussed in the introductory section of this workbook, a key theme within the implementation of personalisation and one of the four domains, presented by the Putting People First Team, as integral to the implementation of personalised approaches.

What is social capital?

'Social capital is generated when people work together to make things happen. It's what's generated when people get involved and ask others to get involved.' (Lyon, 2007)

'...the basic idea of "social capital" is that one's family, friends and associates constitute an important asset, one that can be called upon in a crisis, enjoyed for its own sake and/or leveraged for material gain. (Woolcock, 2001)

Social networks within this understanding are far-reaching and include the full range of contacts and associates that an individual may have. Alongside the ability to identify the full range of contacts and networks that an individual may have to draw upon, communication skills are also a core component of being able to effectively use the social capital that is available.

Different audiences have different levels of understanding and as such, it is necessary to consider how information is conveyed and received. Professional groups, in particular, often use jargon, and this competence acknowledges that there are many ways in which communication can be used and adapted to increase the engagement of different stakeholders.

Activity: Identifying and communicating with social networks

Identifying the whole of an individual's social network involves consideration of daily activities and routines to ensure that all contacts and associations are highlighted. This activity will enable the reader to work through the various contacts an individual may have and the role they play within the social network and possible social capital considerations. This activity can be carried out individually or in a group and related to anyone.

Instructions

- List the various contacts within the person's life.
- State what type of contact this is ie. daily, weekly, monthly, occasionally, face-to-face, telephone, letter, email etc.
- Rank according to importance (1 = very important, 5 = not important at all).

Group	Who?	What type of contact?	Ranking (1 – 5)
Family Immediate and extended family, in-laws, cousins, grandparents etc.			
Friends School friends, work friends, pen pals, anyone else you consider a friend etc.			
Friends and family of friends and family Anyone else you have contact with via others' networks			
Community and neighbourhood Neighbours, shop keepers, faith group members, policeman etc.			
Hobbies and interests Social groups and activities, walking groups, adult education classes, exercise classes etc.			
Professionals GP, practice nurse, health visitors, support workers, social workers, CPN, consultants etc.			
Colleagues and peers Workmates, educational contacts, contacts via support groups or services etc.			
Virtual contacts Discussion forums, bulletin boards, Twitter, Facebook, Myspace, Bebo etc.			
Others Anyone else you may have contact with as part of your regular routine eg. saying hello to the crossing patrol man etc.			

Each person has a wide range of contacts and identification of each of these will provide an overview to the context in which an individual operates. Communication with different stakeholders needs to be flexible, and understanding what roles different individuals and groups play will assist in the communication processes. A service user may not wish to disclose their difficulties to some contacts but will for others, and this must also be considered. It is not always necessary for an individual to be aware of difficulties in order to provide support, this exercise has highlighted a whole spectrum of contacts that a person may have, many of whom are unconnected to the mental health field, and who still represent a significant source of social interaction for the person concerned.

Types of communication

Once the range of an individual's social network has been identified and detailed, consider the following questions for each category of contacts.

- Has the person disclosed their mental health issues to this group/person?
- Are the individuals/groups likely to be aware of mental health issues and what that might mean to someone who is experiencing mental distress? What impact (if any) does this awareness have?
- What communication approach would be most effective for this group? (eg. plain English, visual representations/pictures etc)
- Is there a need for information/psycho-education for any of the contacts in order to assist them to better support the individual?
- What do the individuals/group of contacts contribute to the individual in terms of support? (eg. social contact, emotional support, practical assistance, providing a service etc)

Often an individual suffering mental distress experiences a high degree of social isolation, however, there is usually a range of contacts which are not considered, and these can hold a number of roles and meanings for the person.

By breaking down the person's social network in this way it is possible to achieve an overview of what roles are played, by whom, and also what level of communication is required to maximise the involvement in an individual's life.

Social context in this format allows for the consideration of the full range of social networks. These form the basis of identifying what social capital is available for the individual to draw upon to assist in the development of personalised care and support to meet the presenting needs.

Competence 3

Understand their role and that of others within a multidisciplinary setting.

The introduction of personalised support represents a significant role shift for both service users and workers, as it requires a level of partnership that has not previously been present in mental health or social care. Roles within mental health are often blurred, and the integration of health and social care has further compounded this blurring (Bogg, 2008).

Personalised care and the roles that workers and service users play going forward is a fundamental change in both thinking and culture, as the principles of choice and control. The rough guide published by SCIE in relation to personalised care (Carr, 2008) suggests that social workers in particular could see an increase in creative, person-centred approaches that have not previously been possible within the care management frameworks. Other changes will include social care workers increasingly operating within private arrangements between service users and individuals (for example as personal assistants), and the scope for third sector providers increasing as the market grows to provide the range of choices that service users will need.

Within personalised support the roles that an individual plays is subject to a partnership that places stakeholders on an equal footing. Within this partnership the aspects of choice and control for service users and carers become the central focus. In this context the service user moves from passive recipient to citizen and decision maker, and the worker moves from protection and control and towards partner and enabler. In mental health this may be particularly difficult, and issues such as compulsion under the Mental Health Act and risk aversion need to be addressed and considered if this enhanced partnership is to be achieved within care and support planning.

Activity: Defining roles

There is often confusion between role and title, and this activity aims to assist the reader to identify role by identifying distinct activities and how these activities interact across different stakeholders involved in the provision of support.

Instructions

On a piece of paper clearly identify the task you are mapping, draw at least two boxes on the page (the number of boxes you draw relates to the number of individuals involved in the task you are working through). Break the task down into small steps and identify which individual is responsible for that step. Once the activity has been mapped into the steps add in lines to link the activities together.

Example

Task (simplified example)

To facilitate access to swimming lessons for Service user A, who has difficulty with motivation in starting new tasks, the worker agrees to source local options – five different classes are available.

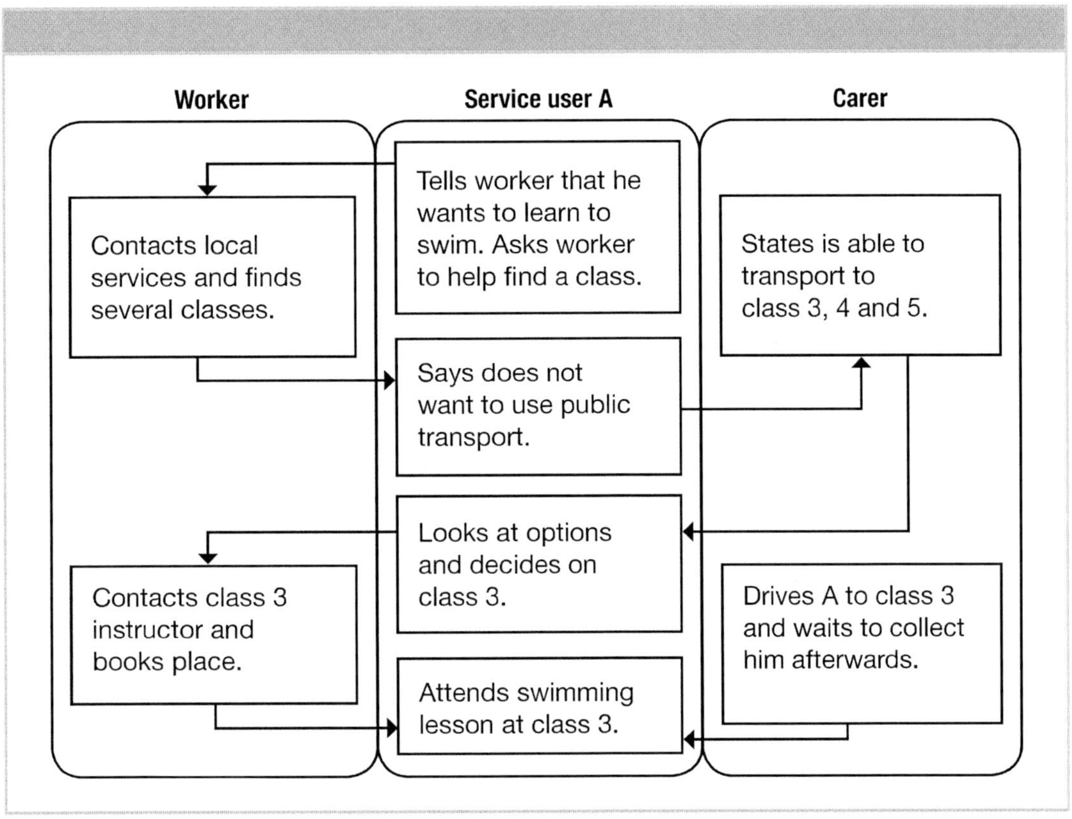

Questions to be considered

In your personal exercise consider the following as you set out your roles and tasks.

- What are the risks involved in the task in which roles are being assigned?
- How can the risks be minimised?
- Are there aspects of the task that the worker is taking on which could be undertaken by the service user and/or carer?
- What are the choices available to the service user/carer in the task identified?

Competence 4

Be able to engage in a collaborative assessment process.

There has been significant evidence and debate within the field over the last decade concerning the need to engage in collaborative assessment and care processes with service users, carers, and other involved parties (Jobes *et al*, 2005; Clarke *et al*, 2009; Rapaport *et al*, 2006; Bee *et al*, 2007), and this is reflected throughout government policy, and inspection and quality standards. Self-assessment is a core theme of the implementation of personalisation, and is an area that is so far developing with varied successes. The white paper, *Our Health, Our Care, Our Say* (DH, 2006) stated that self-assessment was the means of giving people more control over the provision of social care services, and this has been supported in a range of schemes, debates and pilots since this document was published (RiPfA, 2006; Griffiths *et al*, 2005; Unity-Sale, 2008; Henwood & Hudson, 2008).

There has been some resistance and anxiety on the part of professional groups in regard to implementation of self-assessment, and the eligibility framework for receiving social care services adds an additional complexity to this area. Current intentions appear to be that local authorities are looking to integrate self-assessment into the resource allocation schemes as a means of moving forward. This model takes the self-assessment and allocates points in each assessment domain. The higher the need, the higher the points, similar to the previous systems in social housing allocation, and points result in a cash value which determines the entitlement in terms of individual budgetary allocation for each user. While this may be a valid system for determining resources, it can be limiting on the creation of a holistic assessment in mental health.

The social care eligibility framework is focused upon risks to independence in a number of areas, whereas mental health operates within an integrated health and social care environment and spans the full biological, psychological and social spectrum of needs and risks, a difference that has traditionally been difficult to reconcile over the life of integrated services to date. In this context, workers will need to ensure that service users and carers are able to express the full range of needs as they see them, as a core part of the assessment process, and ensure that this does not become limited to what is considered an eligible need.

Reflection exercise

Worker

- How would you need to change your practice to promote self-assessment as the central assessment process?

- What are the benefits of self-assessment, and are there any concerns about self-assessment?

- How would you ensure self-assessment in the assessment and management of risk?

Service user/carer

- How do you think self-assessment will impact upon the care/support you access?

- What are the benefits and concerns, in your view, in regard to basing care package decisions on your self-assessment of needs?

- How do you assess your own risks, and what support would you need to do this?

Competence 5

Acknowledge the part that families and carers play in the service user's support network and be able to engage them as partners in care.

One of the core elements of social work practice has traditionally been to consider the individual in their family context. This is not as evident in other professional groups, however, and it may be that the integration of health and social care has seen a reduction in the systemic approaches that social workers once routinely practised. The focus on carers, and their role in the self-determination and social inclusion agenda, means that workers need to return to this model of thinking and develop competence in identifying social supports and influences within the individual's life.

The role of carers in health and social care has long been recognised as a key protective factor for those experiencing mental distress, with policy and legislation being in place to provide assessment and support services for carers.

In 2008 the current Carer's Strategy was published, setting out the government's 10-year plan to support and develop the carer role, with five aims to be achieved by 2018, these are:

- carers will be respected as expert care partners and will have access to the integrated and personalised services they need to support them in their caring role
- carers will be able to have a life of their own alongside their caring role
- carers will be supported so that they are not forced into financial hardship by their caring role
- carers will be supported to stay mentally and physically well and treated with dignity
- children and young people will be protected from inappropriate caring and have the support they need to learn, develop and thrive, to enjoy positive childhoods and to achieve against all the Every Child Matters outcomes.
  (DH, 2008; p16)

A carer is not necessarily just a person who lives with the service user; carer activities can range from emotional support, to practical assistance, such as transport, domestic tasks and assistance with living skills, to social activities. In families where one (or more) individual (s) has a mental health difficulty, the members that provide support may not identify themselves as carers, and the relationships present may be based on a range of emotional and familial interactions and connections that can impact upon all of the members. Consideration of these factors are a core element of this competency area, and having an awareness of roles and relationships can be useful in terms of the support an individual may have and need to promote recovery in mental health.

Activity: Genograms

There is a number of tools that can be used to look at family systems. This activity introduces the genogram, a type of family tree that helps to create a visual representation of family make-up and relationships.

Instructions

✓ This activity can be carried out either on your own or in discussion between two or more people.
✓ Identify your family members; draw them and the relationships between them on a piece of paper using the following key.

Key to symbols

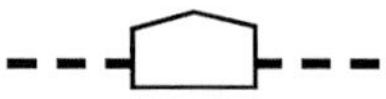 Cohabiting

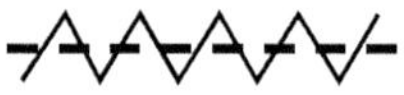 Hostile relationship

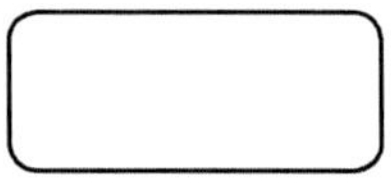 Male

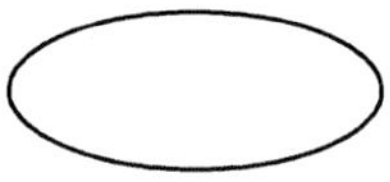 Female

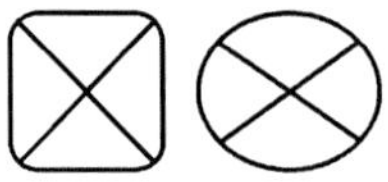 Died (number represents age at death)

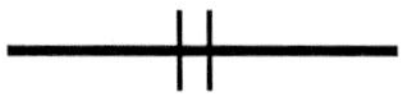 Divorce/separation

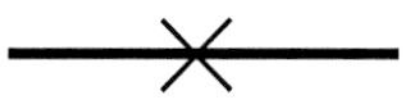 Widowed

Example

Chris is a 19-year-old male; he is the child of second marriages of both his parents. Chris's father is divorced from his first wife, and Chris has two half siblings from his father's first marriage who live with their mother. Chris's mother is a widow from her first marriage, and Chris has three half sisters – one of which died as a young teenager; the other two he lived with throughout his childhood. One of these half sisters from his mother's first marriage lives with Chris's half brother from his father's first marriage. Chris knows both sets of his grandparents, however, his paternal grandparents are now dead. Chris's mother and his father's first wife have a very hostile relationship.

Based on the brief description of Chris's immediate family, his genogram would be:

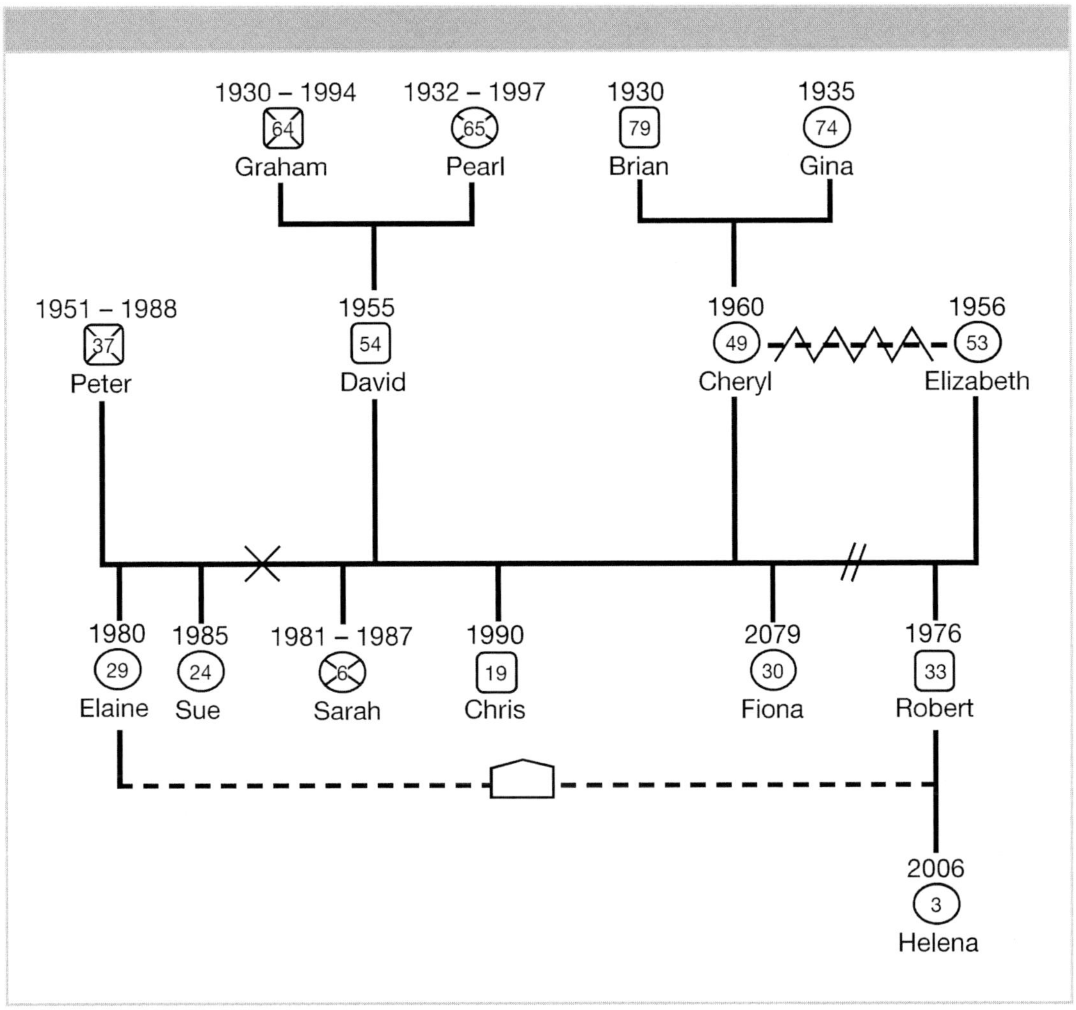

Aunts, uncles, cousins and other extended family can be added to the genogram where the person feels the relationship is significant to their family or social situation. Emotional relationships should be added where they have an impact on the individual or their relationships within the family system.

Competence 6

Be able to communicate across disciplinary, professional and organisational boundaries.

Relationship building and the notion of the therapeutic relationship have been key features in social care, and specifically social work, for many years (Sudbery, 2002; Trevithick, 2003), and communication skills are part of the training courses of most professions.

> *'The communication "bridge" that relationships provide acts as a vital link – or point of human connection – across two worlds: the world of the social worker and the world of the service user, carer or other person.* (SCIE, 2010)

The ability to communicate between worker and service user or carer is a vital element within the personalisation agenda, as the partnership required is far more focused upon the choices and preferences of the user rather than the previous emphasis on professional decisions. To achieve this shift in practice, workers will need to use their skills to advocate, negotiate and inform to ensure the service user and carer are able to exercise their choices.

Skills such as those listed, are essential if personalised care is to be fully implemented.

- Listening – actively to capture another's point of view.
- Language – use of plain English.
- Empathy – hearing and understanding, and conveying this understanding.
- Reflection – reflecting back information, to ensure understanding and give perspective.
- Questioning – obtaining information and stimulating ideas.

While it is vital that these skills are routinely used and applied to the relationship between worker and service user, there is also a need to apply the same level of skill to the relationships between professionals and agencies in order to maximise the partnership potential.

Partnerships between workers and services are necessary, as no one service, or person, will be solely providing the support needed, and in order to prevent misunderstandings and duplication, the services need to be as joined up as possible. To achieve this level of partnership, communication skills on all parts need to be practised. Areas such as information sharing, awareness of the overall context of the individual, and a clear understanding of how each support mechanism impacts upon the individual can all help to provide a more tailored and positive experience. In addition, the relationships between services and professionals are also affected by the differing criteria and functions, and agencies need to be clear regarding their foci and agendas.

Communication skills are core competencies that need to be applied to all interactions. The use of language and the ability to listen and understand differing perspectives all form essential components in implementing the personalisation agenda in mental health. Co-production needs to be further developed in order to ensure that informed choice is available and the ability of services and communities to understand, adapt and partner in providing options, are central to the transformation process.

Reflection exercise

- Do you change your language according to your audience?
  - If so, how and what is the impact?
  - If not, what types of language do you use and how does this affect how others hear you?

- How does hearing jargon from others, which you don't understand, impact upon what you hear and how you feel?

- When talking to another person, what types of behaviour and/or communication, make you feel like you are being listened to?

NB

SCIE online has a selection of e-learning activities for improving communication skills, these are available at: http://www.scie.org.uk/publications/elearning/cs/index.asp

Summary

Section 1 considered the 'Working in partnership' capability as follows:

'Developing and maintaining constructive working relationships with service users, carers, families, colleagues, lay people and wider community networks. Working positively with any tensions created by conflicts of interest or aspirations that may arise between the partners in care.'

The competencies presented have considered a range of skills that are important to the shift towards personalised care in mental health. They have particularly highlighted the importance of partnership and communication between all those involved.

Summary exercise

Write a short summary of what this capability means to you in your context/practice, and then answer the following three questions.

- What have you learnt by completing this section?

- How have you now reached competence in this area?

- What do you need to do to maintain your competence?

References

Bee P, Playle J, Lovell K, Barnes P, Gray R & Keeley P (2007) Service user views and expectations of UK-registered mental health nurses: a systematic review of empirical research. *International Journal of Nursing Studies* **45** (3) 442–457.

Bogg D (2008) *The Integration of Mental Health Social Work and the NHS*. Exeter: Learning Matters.

Carr S (2008) *Personalisation: A Rough Guide*. Adult Services Report 20. London: SCIE.

Clarke SP, Crowe TP, Oades LG & Deane FP (2009) Do goal-setting interventions improve the quality of goals in mental health services? *Psychiatric Rehabilitation Journal* **32** (4) 292–299.

Department of Health (2006) *Our Health, Our Care, Our Say: A new direction for community services*. London: TSO.

Department of Health (2008) *Carers at the Heart of 21st Century Families and Communities: A caring system on your side, a life of your own*. London: TSO.

Finch R (2008) Left holding the cash? *Caring Business* **August** 10.

Gilburt H, Rose D & Slade M (2008) The importance of relationships in mental health care: a qualitative study of service users' experiences of psychiatric hospital admission in the UK. *BMC Health Services Research* [online] **8** 92. Available at: http://www.biomedcentral.com/content/pdf/1472-6963-8-92.pdf (accessed June 2010).

Griffiths P, Harris R & Ullman R (2005) *Self-assessment of health and social care needs by older people: a multimethod systematic review of practices, accuracy, effectiveness and experience.* London: NHS Service Delivery and Organisation R&D Programme.

Henwood M & Hudson B (2008) Individual budgets and personalisation: a new model of integration? *Journal of Integrated Care* **16** (3) 8–16.

Hudson B & Henwood M (2008) *Prevention, Personalisation and Prioritisation in Social Care: Squaring the circle? A report commissioned by CSCI for the review of eligibility criteria* [online]. Available at: http://www.cqc.org.uk/_db/_documents/20080808%20Tracked%20FACS%20Literature%20review_typeset%20v3%20Dom.pdf (accessed June 2010).

Huxley P, Evans S, Bereford P, Davidson B & King S (2009) The principles and provisions of relationships. *Journal of Social Work* **9** (1) 99–117.

Jobes DA, Wong SA, Conrad AK, Drozd JF & Neal-Walden T (2005) The collaborative assessment and management of suicidality versus treatment as usual: a retrospective study with suicidal outpatients. *Suicide and Life-Threatening Behavior* **35** (5) 483–497.

Leadbetter C (2004) *Personalisation through Participation: A new script for public services* [online]. London: Demos. Available at: http://www.demos.co.uk/files/PersonalisationThroughParticipation.pdf (accessed June 2010).

Lyon B (2007) *Social Capital – Observations* [online]. Available at: http://www.social-capital.net/docs/Re-Union%20Case%20Study%202007.pdf (accessed June 2010).

McCabe R & Priebe S (2004) The therapeutic relationship in the treatment of severe mental illness: a review of methods and findings. *International Journal of Social Psychiatry* **50** (2) 115–128.

Office for Disability Issues (2008) *Independent Living: A cross-government strategy about independent living for disabled people*. London: Office for Disability Issues.

Rapaport J, Bellringer S, Pinfold V & Huxley P (2006) Carers and confidentiality in mental health care: considering the role of the carer's assessment: a study of service users', carers' and practitioners' views. *Health and Social Care in the Community* **14** (4) 357–365.

RiPfA (2006) *Self-assessment: How does it work, is it effective and how can it be promoted?* [online]. Available at: http://www.ripfa.org.uk/publications/outlines/outlinesPDF/2.pdf (accessed June 2010).

SCIE (2010) *Forming and Maintaining Relationships with Service Users, Carers, Professionals and Others*. [online] Available at: http://www.scie.org.uk/publications/elearning/cs/cs02/resource/index.html (accessed June 2010).

Shattell M, Starr S & Thomas S (2007) 'Take my hand, help me out', mental health service recipients' experience of the therapeutic relationship. *International Journal of Mental Health Nursing* **16** (4) 274–284.

Sudbery J (2002) Key features of therapeutic social work: the use of relationship. *Journal of Social Work Practice* **16** (2) 149–162.

Trevithick P (2003) Effective relationship-based practice: a theoretical exploration. *Journal of Social Work Practice* **17** (2) 173–186.

Unity-Sale A (2008) Knowing me, knowing you. *Community Care* **7 August** 28–29.

Woolcock M (2001) The place of social capital in understanding social and economic outcomes. *Canadian Journal of Policy Research* **2** (1) 1–17.

Section 2: Respecting diversity

Working in partnership with service users, carers, families and colleagues to provide care and interventions that not only make a positive difference but also do so in ways that respect and value diversity including age, race, culture, disability, gender, spirituality and sexuality.

The concept of culturally competent services, and practice has received significant attention over the past decade with a range of definitions. One definition, which was compiled from a range of research evidence, was outlined by RiPfA in 2008; they stated that cultural competence meant:

> *'... how well an organisation and the individuals within it provide care to people with diverse values, beliefs and behaviours. This can involve designing services to meet social, cultural and language needs. It means valuing individuals, families, communities and protecting their dignity. Knowledge about diversity is turned into specific standards, policies, practices and attitudes. These help to improve the quality of services and produce better outcomes for everybody.'* (RiPfA, 2008 p1)

Aims

This section of the workbook will consider the area of equality and diversity in terms of a personalised approach and support system. The aims of this section are:

- to consider personalisation within an equality framework
- to consider the impact of culture on choice, control and expectations
- to link culturally competent practice with the implementation of personalised care.

Overview

The population of England and Wales is becoming increasingly diverse, and when considering changes to a public service system there needs to be an awareness of the different cultural groups that may access health and social care services and the diversity of the needs they may have.

10 areas of competence are included within this second shared capability, these are:

Competence 1: Understand and acknowledge diversity relating to age, gender, race culture, disability, spirituality and sexuality.

Competence 2: Understand the impact of discrimination and prejudice on mental health and mental health services.

Competence 3:	Demonstrate a commitment to equal opportunities for all persons and encourage their active participation in every aspect of care and treatment.
Competence 4:	Respond to the needs of people sensitively with regard to all aspects of diversity.
Competence 5:	Demonstrate the ability to promote people's rights and responsibilities and recognise the service user's rights to privacy, dignity, respect and confidentiality.
Competence 6:	Demonstrate the ability to work as a member of the therapeutic team to contribute to evidence-based programmes of care and treatment that are sensitive to diversity.
Competence 7:	Provide care and treatment that recognises the importance of housing, employment, occupational opportunities, recreational activities, advocacy, social networks and welfare benefits.
Competence 8:	Demonstrate adherence to local, professional and national codes of practice.
Competence 9:	Demonstrate effective knowledge of organisational policies and practices to maintain the role and the capacity of the therapeutic team to provide evidence-based care that is sensitive to diversity.
Competence 10:	Demonstrate a commitment to active participation in clinical supervision and lifelong learning.

By working through these competencies within this section the reader will begin to apply the personalisation approach to a framework of equality and diversity.

Values and social care have traditionally been linked, and the personalisation of care has the potential to increase competence in responding to diversity as the service user and carer voice becomes central to support services in a way that has not previously been the case.

Competence 1

Understand and acknowledge diversity relating to age, gender, race, culture, disability, spirituality and sexuality.

Diversity in its basic form means difference, and people's differences can be many and varied. The six streams of diversity are each huge areas in their own rights, and the interaction between them can mean that complex combinations inform and shape an individual's cultural perspective and understanding. Behaviours, beliefs and expectations all have an impact upon how an individual experiences a service or an approach, and it is the worker's role to be aware of these when communicating, assessing and planning with an individual (and their family) how to provide the support they may need.

A range of issues needs to be considered within the diversity context, these can include areas such as:

- accessibility – physical and emotional; including environment accessibility; opening times and flexibility; child care responsibilities; location and identification with the building; transport issues
- appropriate treatment – physical and emotional; is the environment appropriate for the needs; does the treatment and support take account of, and respond to, needs, beliefs, behaviours and cultural norms
- prejudice and stigma – workers and service users are as susceptible to prejudicial views as the general population; views held about certain groups; certain needs; certain professions/services, and what an individual believes about them, all have an impact on the level of engagement with, and the effectiveness of, any support accessed.
- additional support needs – arising from either the diversity of need or the response of services as a result of the need.

Case studies

The following case studies are examples of some of the projects that have been introduced across the country. (Full details and further examples are presented by the Department of Health [online])

East Midlands

200 individuals from local black and minority ethnic (BME) communities have been trained by one NHS mental health trust in wellness and recovery/resilience action planning (WRAP). This includes people from the African-Caribbean, Bangladeshi and Somali communities, members of the gypsy and Irish travelling communities and carers and service users from the Irish community. Those who have been trained are working with their communities and mental health services – providing support to individuals to develop their personal well-being plans. Evaluations, to date, are showing high levels of satisfaction and impact with this approach.

South west

One primary care trust (PCT) joined forces with a range of public bodies and agencies and held joint consultation events on disability and gender issues. The idea was that on one day the community and voluntary sector groups and networks could talk to all the public authorities with a duty to develop disability and gender equality schemes.

North west

Three local agencies have linked with the local university to promote a better understanding of the needs of older lesbian, gay, bisexual and transgender (LGBT) people in service provision. This includes health care, social care, housing, transport and other services across the public sector. An older people's LGBT group has written *Moving Forward* – a training and resource pack for public sector agencies, published by Salford University in October 2007.

South west

Individuals who were on the caseload of one BME mental health team were asked if they would like to work as volunteers. Three were recruited in March 2008 and are now working as part of the team.

Question to consider

- What activities are happening in your area, which contribute to the overall understanding of equality and diversity issues?

Competence 2

Understand the impact of discrimination and prejudice on mental health and mental health services.

Stigma and prejudice are key areas within mental health. The label of mental health service user carries a number of meanings – both in how the individual understands themself, and also how services and society view and respond to them. In a society where one in four of us will experience a mental health problem at some time in our lives, it is still the case that the terms 'mental illness' and 'mental health problem' raise a number of fears within members of the wider public.

Media representation of mental ill health remains sensationalised, with papers carrying stories of homicide and suicide to the exclusion of any positive examples. There has been significant research into the impact of discrimination and prejudice on mental well-being (Sayce, 2001; Pinfold *et al*, 2005; Schneider & Bramley, 2008; Morgan *et al*, 2007; Curran *et al*, 2007), and it is shown that negative attitudes are a barrier to recovery from mental health problems. It is well recognised that social interaction and social context can influence a person's level of distress and their chances of recovering, and as such, these views need to be considered and challenged.

Personalised care emphasises social involvement as the key to service delivery and design, with community groups and informal support playing a significant role in providing support. The whole person approach involves understanding the full range of influences and aspects of a person's life.

Considering the range of support services that a person may access is an important activity within the personalisation approach. Choice and control extend much wider than just health and social care, and the social inclusion and recovery approaches in mental health include a range of activities that are part of normal daily life. Mainstream services, community involvement and social networks, such as friends and family, all have a part to play, and the discriminating social attitudes to those experiencing mental health problems have the potential to place barriers in the way of the social involvement needed.

As a result of prejudice and stereotyping, individuals who are seen as having a mental health problem can find themselves excluded from certain areas of their communities, and this can have a significant impact on the choices available.

Possible social supports

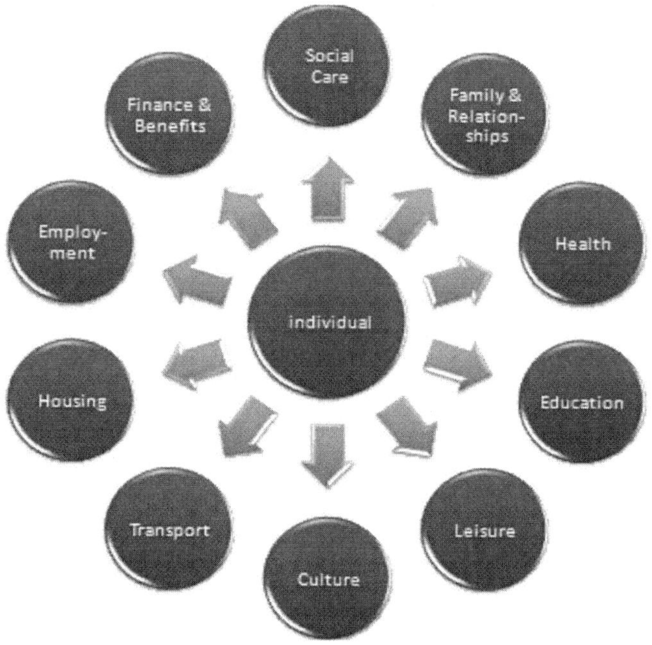

This illustration is not complete and there are many other groups and activities that a person may take part in. The prejudice and discrimination that a person with a mental health difficulty can experience is largely as a result of fear and misinformation, yet it is an issue that can affect anyone, and there is a range of projects that have been set up to challenge the stigma and discrimination associated with mental health problems.

Case study

Time to Change

A range of projects have been set up with a number of organisations including MIND, Rethink and Mental Health Media, with funding from the Big Lottery Fund and Comic Relief. All aim to challenge the stigma associated with mental health and provide information and education.

Work includes:

- local community projects
- a national high-profile media campaign
- a mass-participation physical activity week
- training for student doctors and teachers.

Competence 3

Demonstrate a commitment to equal opportunities for all persons and encourage their active participation in every aspect of care and treatment.

Service user involvement is a significant focus within mental health services, and the move towards personalised care emphasises a level of partnership that has not previously been evident within treatment. Co-production between services and service users and carers is a development that supports equal opportunities as it places the service user as central to the process and an equal partner in the care process.

Equality does not mean the same; differences are just as important as similarities. Different people come with different needs, skills and strengths, however, opportunities and access to services, supports and experiences are the areas that need to be supported in order to achieve equality. The Equality Bill, which was presented to the House of Commons in April 2009, places a legislative framework around the equality and diversity framework and will place a duty on organisations to respond to individuals in a way that ensures equality and fairness and challenges discrimination where it occurs.

Worker and service user presumptions can be an issue within the delivery of care that promotes equality and involvement. As with wider society, the mental health system has a culture of its own, one that is based on perceptions of risk, familiarity with how things have previously been, professional cultures that are based on a power dynamic which 'does to' rather than 'does with', and social prejudices and stereotypes of what having a mental health problem means. All of these areas are challengeable and can change in nature and over time. However, it is necessary to be aware that culture is a powerful thing, and system change can take time to achieve.

As already stated, stereotyping and prejudice can create barriers for mental health service users in terms of what support systems they can access and how they experience social situations. The task in this competence is to challenge attitudes that result in exclusion or rejection from social opportunities or experiences, and support individuals to experience the full range of social and community options as part of their support plans.

In terms of mental health treatment itself, the individual should be central to all the planning processes. Assessment, care planning, and risk management are all key aspects of mental health care and practitioners should undertake these aspects in partnership with service users and carers. This is a shift from the previous practices, which were based on professional views of what should happen (Glennister, 1994; Barnes & Shardlow, 1997; Warne & McAndrew, 2007). The work of Beresford and colleagues (Beresford & Branfield, 2006; Beresford & Campbell, 1994; Beresford & Croft, 2004), as well as many others, has considered empowerment within services, and it has been shown that involvement and empowerment have positive outcomes in terms of promoting recovery.

Exercise

Consider the questions below in the context of mental health services. This can be as a practitioner or as a service user/carer of mental health services. The role you play affects how you experience the service.

- How do you support equal opportunities and equal access within your practice? What types of actions, behaviours or attitudes have you experienced or practised?

or

- Can you think of examples of when you have accessed services and have felt that the opportunities available to you, in terms of care options, have been the same or different from what is available to other people?

- How do you involve service users and carers in assessment and care planning? What type of activities or interactions have you been involved in?

or

- How involved within care planning and assessment do you feel and what makes you feel this way?

We are all service users of some types of services, whether this is with a GP or other physical health service, or local authority services such as housing, employment, benefits or education. It can be helpful to reflect on how you feel being a service user in other areas and compare those experiences to the mental health care system.

- As a service user or carer of any service do you feel involved in care and treatment decisions? What helps you to feel that way?

Competence 4

Respond to the needs of people sensitively with regard to all aspects of diversity.

A person's cultural context and understanding defines their behaviour, the decisions they make and the risks they are willing to take, and as such, within service delivery, staff need to be aware of, and be sensitive to the cultural and social norms of the individual. Language, beliefs, behaviour and values are all aspects that shape how a person responds and how they interact with others.

There has been significant emphasis on race within mental health, including the Delivering Race Equality (DRE) programme, which is a response to a number of high profile cases, including the death of David 'Rocky' Bennett. The emphasis of the programme is to improve the experience of BME groups within the mental health system and acknowledgement that different groups have different needs that need to be considered and responded to.

The vision for the DRE programme (DH, 2005)

By 2010 the mental health system will be characterised by:

- less fear of mental health services among BME communities and service users
- increased satisfaction with services
- a reduction in the rate of admission of people from BME communities to psychiatric inpatient units
- a reduction in the disproportionate rates of compulsory detention of BME service users in inpatient units
- fewer violent incidents that are secondary to inadequate treatment of mental illness
- a reduction in the use of seclusion in BME groups
- the prevention of deaths in mental health services following physical intervention
- more BME service users reaching self-reported states of recovery
- a reduction in the ethnic disparities found in prison populations
- a more balanced range of effective therapies, such as peer support services and psychotherapeutic and counselling treatments, as well as pharmacological interventions that are culturally appropriate and effective
- a more active role for BME communities and BME service users in the training of professionals, in the development of mental health policy, and in the planning and provision of services
- a workforce and organisation capable of delivering appropriate and responsive mental health services to BME communities.

While race is an important consideration, when thinking about equality and diversity there are a number of strands that need to be considered, these are:

- race
- religion and beliefs

- sexuality
- gender
- age
- disability.

Each of the strands has equal importance and services need to respond in a sensitive manner to the needs that may arise as a result of any of these areas. Many of the aims of the DRE programme should be extended to the other areas. This would assist in the increase in ability of the mental health system to respond to diverse and multiple needs, and improve the service user experience by being sensitive to the full range of an individual's experience.

Each strand of the diversity framework has the potential to experience exclusion from wider society, this can be as a result of direct discrimination based on fear, misunderstanding or negative attitudes, or as a result of indirect discrimination, which largely arises as a result of not taking account of additional or different needs and understandings that result.

From a personalisation perspective the 'whole-person' approach is the key, and this is important for an individual's understanding of themselves and their cultural context, and as such can impact upon how the person feels about the service and also the effectiveness of any treatment package that is delivered. From initial assessment through to detailed care planning and review processes, the diversity of the individual must be considered. Interactions, reactions and responses are all shaped by how the individual experiences themselves and their surroundings, and as such, the worker's task is to make sure that the whole context is taken into account.

Questions to consider

- How can the aims of the DRE programme be applied to the other areas eg. sexuality or disability?
- How would this improve service user experience of the system and make services more sensitive to diverse needs?
- How could a lack of sensitivity to these issues affect support choices?

Competence 5

Demonstrate the ability to promote people's rights and responsibilities and recognise the service user's rights to privacy, dignity, respect and confidentiality.

Human rights and equality and diversity are all linked agendas, the basis of all public services, including mental health, is that individual rights are observed at all times. The additional rights that are in place under other legislation, such as the Disability Discrimination Act (2005), the Mental Capacity Act (2005) and the Mental Health Act (1983) (as amended by the Mental Health Act (2007)), support these and anyone working within public services has a duty to ensure that the individual's rights are upheld.

Human rights legislation covers a range of rights that individuals have in relation to privacy, dignity, confidentiality and respect.

Article 3: Prohibition of torture

No one shall be subjected to torture or to inhuman or degrading treatment or punishment. This means that detention and treatment within mental health services cannot be used as punishment. The mental health system is based on evidence-based treatment that must include consultation and involvement with the service user and consent should always be sought, however, it is possible to treat without consent if the situation warrants it.

Article 5: The right to liberty

Everyone has the right to liberty and security of person. No one shall be deprived of his liberty, save in the following cases and in accordance with a procedure prescribed by law. This allows for the lawful detention of persons of unsound mind. The Mental Health Act is the framework for which this can occur. However, everyone who is deprived of his liberty by arrest or detention is entitled to take proceedings by which the lawfulness of his detention can be determined. This includes a right of appeal and review by an independent tribunal.

Article 8: The right to respect for family and private life

Everyone has the right to respect for his or her private and family life, home and correspondence. Within the mental health system this includes the privacy and dignity agenda, whereby private spaces and confidentiality of information must be upheld. Issues such as sexuality are protected under this article, and services have a duty to respect choices made by service users.

It should be noted that privacy and confidentiality within services is not an absolute right. There are circumstances when information must be shared, this is related to harm – either to self, others or children, and workers within the field need to make sure that service users are aware of these circumstances.

Article 14: Prohibition of discrimination

Rights and freedoms are in place without discrimination on any ground such as sex, race, colour, language, religion, political or other opinion, national or social origin, association with a national minority, property, birth or other status. This article protects the equality and diversity strands discussed in the previous competence and also supports equality of opportunity, making it contrary to human rights to discriminate against any individual or group on the basis of diversity.

Article 17: Prohibition of the abuse of rights

This article protects the rights that are set down by making it unlawful to abuse any of the rights that an individual has.

The responsibility and duty to uphold these rights is placed upon all public services, which include health and social care providers, and there are legal sanctions available when discrimination occurs – these include tribunals and the courts as well as mediation services. Personalisation does not deviate from this duty, however, it will expand it as different types of providers and more community and informal support is available.

The Mental Health Act (as amended) code of practice (DH, 2008a) has a direct link to these rights and responsibilities, especially in regard to privacy, dignity, respect and confidentiality. The principles guide any action taken under the Mental Health Act, and workers must provide evidence that they have considered these areas within any assessment or treatment process. These help to support the individual's rights in circumstances that could be seen as restrictive and in opposition with the person's wishes and preferences.

Purpose principle

Decisions under the Act must be taken with a view to minimising the undesirable effects of mental disorder, by maximising the safety and well-being (mental and physical) of patients, promoting their recovery and protecting other people from harm.

Least restriction principle

People taking action without a patient's consent must attempt to keep the restrictions they impose on the patient's liberty to a minimum, having regard to the purpose for which the restrictions are imposed.

Respect principle

People taking decisions under the act must recognise and respect the diverse needs, values and circumstances of each patient, including their race, religion, culture, gender, age, sexual orientation and disability. They must consider the patient's views, wishes and feelings (whether expressed at the time or in advance), and follow those wishes wherever practicable and consistent with the purpose of the decision. There must be no unlawful discrimination.

Participation principle

Patients must be given the opportunity to be involved, as far as is practicable in the circumstances, in planning, developing and reviewing their own treatment. The involvement of carers, family members and other people who have an interest in the patient's welfare should be encouraged (unless there are particular reasons to the contrary) and their views taken seriously.

Effectiveness, efficiency and equity principle (resources principle)

People taking decisions under the act must seek to use the resources available to them and to patients in the most effective, efficient and equitable way, to meet the needs of patients and achieve the purpose for which the decision was taken.

This framework helps to support and promote human rights within the mental health setting, and locates the person's rights as central to the process.

Compulsive treatment under the Mental Health Act is one of the most restrictive options available within the health and social care system, and as such, there is a range of safeguards in place that professionals must ensure are upheld. This starts from the process of initial assessment, and mechanisms such as appeal rights, reviews and second opinion doctors all serve to monitor the situation and ensure an individual's rights are maintained.

Case study exercise

Read the following case study and consider the questions below.

A referral has been received for a Mental Health Act assessment from a GP regarding Susan, a 38-year-old woman who is married with two children (aged six and 15). She is well known to services and her mother, Sylvia, is involved in caring for both Susan and the two children.

Susan is diagnosed with bipolar disorder and has had at least one previous admission when she became paranoid and shouted at a local shop assistant who she believed was following her. The GP feels that Susan is very anxious, has told him that she is hearing voices talking about her and has expressed thoughts about hurting her husband.

Susan and her husband have frequent arguments, and the police have been called to the address on two occasions as a result. One visit involved Frank being taken to the police station on a charge of assault against Susan. He returned home the following day and Susan did not press charges. The couple have been together for 10 years and Frank is the father of the six-year-old, it is not clear whether the 15-year-old has contact with her father.

Susan is of Irish origin, and she is a devout catholic and heavily involved in the local church. Frank is British and does not have any religious affiliation. Susan talks regularly to her local priest. The priest's view is that she is not having psychotic episodes but is having religious experiences. Susan agrees that this is the case and believes that her previous admission was as a result of her actions being misunderstood.

Questions

- What aspects of diversity need to be considered?

- What rights does Susan have at this point?

- What rights do Sylvia, Frank and the two children have at this point?

- What are the confidentiality issues in the case?

- What are the actions that need to be taken?

- What are the possibilities for personalised care in this case?

Competence 6

Demonstrate the ability to work as a member of the therapeutic team to contribute to evidence-based programmes of care and treatment that are sensitive to diversity.

Each area of an individual's life and each professional group brings with it a distinct perspective and evidence base, and the benefit of multidisciplinary approaches is based on these differences. Therapeutic approaches within a personalisation context are not limited to formal therapy, but rather relate to the ways in which interactions and interventions can be used to promote recovery and increased social functioning and inclusion.

Competence in this area relates to the ability of the individual to express their perspective and evidence base to ensure that the care and support takes account of the whole person. Self-directed care is an approach that is based within the social model of disability, promoting choice and control for the service user as both a way to improve service delivery and also as a method of supporting the recovery process. Health, social care and community supports all have a role and a voice in the process, as each element provides a piece of the recovery jigsaw and plays an important part in understanding the context in which the individual operates.

Possible influences within a service user's social context

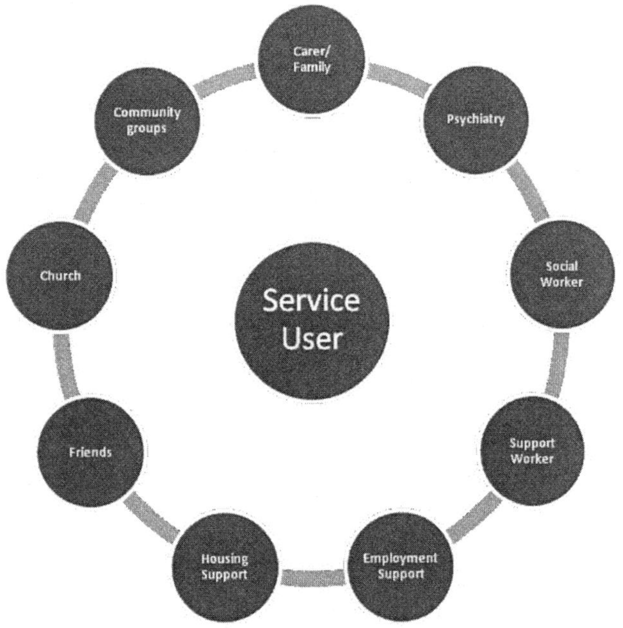

Competence 7

Provide care and treatment that recognises the importance of housing, employment, occupational opportunities, recreational activities, advocacy, social networks and welfare benefits.

As discussed in competence 2, the individual's whole social situation needs to be considered within the personalised approach. This perspective is rooted in the social model of disability, which considers the wider context of a person (Burchardt, 2004; Finklestein, 1980; Oliver & Barnes, 1998). Mental health is not just about a collection of symptoms or behaviours and how these are treated; to have such a narrow focus limits the effectiveness of any intervention, and also discounts the strengths and resources of the individual.

Care planning within the social context needs to account for the full range of social experiences that the individual has and can draw upon, and this is explicit within the personalisation agenda (DH, 2008b).

Exercise

Using the following case study, develop an initial care plan, taking account of all the circumstances of the situation. Imagine James is living in your area and draw upon the resources that are locally available to construct the plan.

James is a 23-year-old, African-Caribbean man, he lives alone in a one bedroom flat in a town centre. He was a student at university studying graphic design until six months ago when he became withdrawn and anxious and felt unable to continue with his course. Over the last six months he has rarely left his flat, his friends and family have been concerned about him but have not had very much contact in this time. Prior to this situation James was very active; he enjoyed sports and live music, and was a member of the local cycling club. He considers himself spiritual, but is not affiliated with any particular church or religion. James' student loan is no longer available to him, and he has not felt able to go to the job centre in this time and so has not claimed any benefits. He is behind with his rent, and his landlord is now threatening to evict him if the situation is not resolved. He has given him four weeks. He is also in debt to credit card companies and has been avoiding his bills.

James has been referred to your service by his GP at the request of his mum. He is willing to see a worker but only on a home visit as he feels unable to come into the centre. He has not previously been known to services and has no mental health history prior to this episode.

Competence 8

Demonstrate adherence to local, professional and national codes of practice.

The Mental Health Act code of practice has already been discussed within this section under competence 5, and workers and services need to remain mindful of the guiding principles set out in all of their duties, as is the case with the human rights (competence 5) and equality and diversity frameworks (competence 4) that have been presented.

Professional codes of practice are in place for each professional group, and within these the focus on service user involvement, rights and self-determination is present. Personalised care supports the aims of each of the codes of practice and workers should always ensure that such codes are observed in all of the activities and professional relationships.

Exercise

In relation to your own professional code of practice, consider the following questions.

- What are the core principles of the code of practice for your professional group?

- How do you evidence your adherence to these principles and codes? Give at least three examples from your own practice or activities.

  Personalisation supports the following principles:

  - service user involvement
  - creativity in support options
  - choice
  - empowerment
  - self-determination
  - whole-person approaches
  - social interactions and context
  - respect for diversity
  - equality of opportunity and access.

How does your code of practice support these aims?

How do you demonstrate these areas in your practice environment?

Competence 9

Demonstrate effective knowledge of organisational policies and practices to maintain the role and the capacity of the therapeutic team to provide evidence-based care that is sensitive to diversity.

Organisational policies and practice vary across services. However, all providers are required to have equal opportunity policies, equality and diversity schemes and operating policies.

In all aspects of equality and diversity, mental health care and personalisation you are operating within an organisational context. As discussed in competence 3, services also have a culture, and the organisational culture is an important consideration within this competence. These are unique to organisations and are based upon historical development of the service, custom and practice, workforce and leadership characteristics, demographics of the area in which they operate and the status and function of the organisation. While there are overriding duties placed on all services, how these are interpreted and delivered can vary and the practitioner needs to be aware of these factors and how they influence practice.

Exercise

Read your organisation's equality and diversity scheme, equal opportunity policy and the operational policy for your service, then consider the following.

How is this translated into the practice environment?

How does your organisation support equality and diversity in the population it serves?

How explicit are human rights in your organisation's practice policies?

In your team or service practice, how do you observe equality and diversity principles?

What services are available to support equality and diversity? (for example, access to interpreters, advocacy services, groups)

If your organisation provides equality and diversity training, complete this and then again ask yourself the questions above.

Competence 10

Demonstrate a commitment to active participation in clinical supervision and lifelong learning.

Personalisation is a new agenda, however, it is not a new approach and self-determination, choice, control and involvement for service users and carers are all areas that have been embedded within health and social care over the last decade. With this in mind, complete the following exercise in relation to your own continuing professional development activities and needs.

Exercise

Reflect upon the information and activities within section 2 and complete the following SWOT analysis of your skills, knowledge and experience based upon the competencies presented.

Strengths What are your strengths in regard to skills and knowledge of equality and diversity frameworks and how these can be applied to personalised approaches?	**Weaknesses** What are the areas that you need to develop in terms of skills, knowledge or experience to be able to feel fully competent in the area of respecting diversity?
Opportunities What is in place to support your skills and knowledge in terms of a sensitive approach to diversity issues? eg. training availability, reflective supervision, available resources, experiences of colleagues etc	**Threats** What barriers exist within your own practice or your organisational context that could prevent you from taking part in or being able to fully observe equality and diversity principles or implementing personalised care?

For each activity you have undertaken complete the following log.

Date	Activity	Objectives	Reflection	Follow-up
When did you take part and what was the duration of the activity.	What was the activity you completed eg. training, reading, shadowing, supervision discussion etc.	What were the aims and objectives of the activity?	Where the aims and objectives met? What did you learn and how does this inform your current practice?	What are the follow-up actions or learning that you need as a result of this activity?

Summary

The overall capability that has been considered within this section is 'respecting diversity', which means:

> *'Working in partnership with service users, carers, families and colleagues to provide care and interventions that not only make a positive difference but also do so in ways that respect and value diversity including age, race, culture, disability, gender, spirituality and sexuality.'*

The competencies presented have considered a range of skills that are important to the shift towards personalised care in mental health, and have particularly highlighted the role that equality, diversity and human rights play within the process of personalised care. In order to achieve service user focused services that take account of the whole person and their views, beliefs and experiences, the range of diverse needs and understandings must be accounted for within the process.

Summary exercise

Write a short summary of what this capability means to you in your context/practice, and then answer the following three questions.

- What have you learnt by completing this section?

- How have you now reached competence in this area?

- What do you need to do to maintain your competence?

References

Barnes M & Shardlow P (1997) From passive recipient to active citizen: participation in mental health user groups. *Journal of Mental Health* **6** (3) 289–300.

Beresford P & Branfield F (2006) Developing inclusive partnerships: user-defined outcomes, networking and knowledge – a case study. *Health and Social Care in the Community* **14** (5) 436–444.

Beresford P & Campbell J (1994) Disabled people, service users, user involvement and representation. *Disability & Society* **9** (3) 315–325.

Beresford P & Croft S (2004) Service users and practitioners reunited: the key component for social work reform. *British Journal of Social Work* **34** 53–68.

Burchardt T (2004) Capabilities and disability: the capabilities framework and the social model of disability. *Disability and Society* **19** (7) 735–751.

Curran C, Burxgardt T, Knapp M, McDaid D & Li B (2007) Challenges in multidisciplinary systematic reviewing: a study on social exclusion and mental health policy. *Social Policy and Administration* **41** (3) 289–312.

Department of Health (2005) *Delivering Race Equality in Mental Health Care: An action plan for reform inside and outside of services and the government's response to the independent inquiry into the death of David Bennett*. London: TSO.

Department of Health (2008a) *Mental Health Act 1983: Code of Practice*. London: TSO.

Department of Health (2008b) *Putting People First: The whole story* [online]. London: DH. Available at: http://www.dh.gov.uk/en/Publicationsandstatistics/Publications/PublicationsPolicyAndGuidance/DH_089665 (accessed June 2010).

Finkelstein V (1980) *Attitudes and Disabled People: Issues for discussion*. New York: World Rehabilitation Fund.

Glennister D (1994) Patient participation in psychiatric services: a literature review and proposal for a research strategy. *Journal of Advanced Nursing* **19** (4) 802–811.

Morgan C, Burns T, Fitzpatrick R, Pinfold V & Priebe S (2007) Social exclusion and mental health: conceptual and methodological review. *British Journal of Psychiatry* **191** 477–483.

Oliver M & Barnes C (1998) *Disabled People and Social Policy: From exclusion to inclusion* London: Longman.

Pinfold V, Byrne P & Toulmin H (2005) Challenging stigma and discrimination in communities: a focus group study identifying UK mental health service users' main campaign priorities. *International Journal of Social Psychology* **51** (2) 128–138.

RiPfA (2008) *How Can We Ensure Culturally Competent Services?* Outline 14 [online]. Available at: http://www.etn.leeds.ac.uk/document/resources/RPFA_Outline_14.pdf (accessed June 2010).

Sayce L (2001) Social inclusion and mental health. *Psychiatric Bulletin* **25** 121–123.

Schnieder J & Bramley CJ (2008) Towards social inclusion in mental health? *Advances in Psychiatric Treatment* **14** 131–138.

Warne T & McAndrew S (2007) Passive patient or engaged expert? Using a Ptolemaic approach to enhance mental health nurse education and practice. *International Journal of Mental Health Nursing* **16** (4) 224–229.

Section 3: Practising ethically

Recognising the rights and aspirations of service users and their families, acknowledging power differentials and minimising them whenever possible. Providing treatment and care that is accountable to service users and carers within the boundaries prescribed by national (professional), legal and local codes of ethical practice.

Ethics within mental health have been extensively debated, with two branches of ethical thought being applied; these are teleology, which states that the end justifies the means, and deontology, which states that the means are just as important as the eventual outcome (Macdonald & Beck-Dudley, 1994; Bloch & Green, 2006).

The perspective taken varies greatly across the field, and is dependent upon role, context and circumstance. One example could be that a psychiatrist may prescribe a certain medication or intervention that may have negative side effects but which has an evidence-based outcome – this would be a teleological approach. The service user perspective in this situation could be that the negative side effects are not tolerable and as such, they are unwilling to engage, regardless of the outcome as, for them, the negatives of the means outweigh the positive of the ends; this would be deontological. The focus of personalisation is for people to control their lives and manage their own mental health to the greatest possible extent, and this creates a real shift in how practice is viewed, minimising the power dynamics between worker and service user, and emphasising individual rights above all else.

Aims

Section 3 will consider the area of ethical practice in terms of a personalised approach and support system. The aims of this section are:

- to consider personalisation within an ethical perspective
- to apply ethical perspectives to service delivery
- to question decision making against a framework of ethics and values.

Overview

Power and empowerment are key considerations within mental health services, and the development of personalised approaches, which promote choice, control and power sharing, present a challenge to more traditional service approaches. By working through these competencies the reader will be encouraged to consider ethics and values within the practice context and develop their own competency in each area.

Ten areas of competence are included within this third shared capability, these are:

Competence 1:	An understanding of and commitment to the legal and human rights of service users and carers.
Competence 2:	An understanding of the service user's wider social and support networks and the contribution made by carers, family and friends to the recovery process.
Competence 3:	The ability to respond to the needs of people in an ethical, honest, non-judgemental manner.
Competence 4:	The ability to encourage active choices and participation in care and treatment.
Competence 5:	The ability to conduct a legal, ethical and accountable practice that remains open to the scrutiny of peers and colleagues.
Competence 6:	The ability to promote service users' (and carers') rights and responsibilities and recognise and maintain their rights to privacy, dignity, safety, effective treatment and care based on the principle of informed consent.
Competence 7:	The ability to work as a member of the therapeutic team in making a safe and effective contribution to the de-escalation and management of anger and violence especially through the use of control and restraint techniques.
Competence 8:	Adherence to local and professionally prescribed codes of ethical conduct and practice.
Competence 9:	Knowledge of policies, practices and procedures concerning the local implementation of mental health and related legislation.
Competence 10:	The ability to work within the boundaries of local complaints management systems.

By working through the competencies within this section the reader will begin to apply the personalisation approach to an ethical framework.

Competence 1

An understanding of and commitment to the legal and human rights of service users and carers.

The Human Rights Act (HRA) (1998) sets out a range of rights for the individual. These are the rights and freedoms that belong to all of us all of the time (from cradle to grave) and they cannot be 'taken away' from us but they can be claimed, fulfilled or limited in certain circumstances. Human rights protect us by placing public authorities under a duty of care to treat us with fairness, respect, equality, dignity and autonomy (FREDA principles) and setting basic standards which public authorities must adhere to. They also regulate the relationship between public authorities (the State, NHS, social services, police, courts, local authorities etc.) and ordinary citizens.

Articles of the Human Rights Act (HRA) relevant to the personalised approach

There are 18 articles that provide protection for the individual's rights and these are detailed within the HRA (1998). The articles listed here are considered to be those which help to promote an individual's choice, control and preferences and hence directly support the individual's right within a personalised approach.

Article 5 – The right to liberty and security
Article 8 – The right to respect for private and family life
Article 9 – Freedom of thought, conscience and religion
Article 10 – Freedom of expression
Article 14 – Prohibition of discrimination
Article 17 – Prohibition of abuse of rights

The Equality Act (2010) makes the human rights principles of fairness, respect, equality, dignity and autonomy a requirement of services' access and delivery, and this means that support providers need to take a human rights based approach to equality and diversity. This is monitored by the Equality and Human Rights Commission, which has a duty under the Equality Act to monitor progress towards the development of a society in which:

- people's ability to achieve their potential is not limited by prejudice or discrimination
- there is respect for and protection of each individual's human rights
- there is respect for the dignity and worth of each individual
- each individual has an equal opportunity to participate in society
- there is mutual respect between groups based on understanding and valuing of diversity and on shared respect for equality and human rights.

Case study exercise

A mental health team at a local authority has a policy of providing support to service users who want to participate in social activities. Steve, who is gay, asked if a support worker could accompany him to a gay pub. His support worker is uncomfortable with this and suggests an alternative pub to go to.

- Does the support worker have the right to deny Steve his human rights to participate in public life as a gay man?

- Which articles of the HRA are relevant in considering this?

Within a personalised approach the HRA is a framework which supports the diversity and rights of individuals, and means that the choices and options available to a person must consider the whole person and the needs, wishes and strengths they may have.

Competence 2

An understanding of the service user's wider social and support networks and the contribution made by carers, family and friends to the recovery process.

Social approaches to mental health form the basis of many other approaches, and understanding this model is a core element of personalisation. Medical approaches on their own are not enough and there needs to be consideration of the person and their context, as well as treatment of any symptoms (Tew *et al*, 2002; Beresford, 2002; Duggan *et al,* 2002; Bogg, 2008). For recovery to happen there needs to be an awareness of the wider context and social network, and how these impact upon the individual's well-being as well as treatment of the condition.

The social approach to mental distress has evolved from the social model of disability, which views social response to a person's impairment as the disabling factor, with exclusion and discrimination having a direct negative impact on the person's health and well-being.

> *'...disability is understood as an unequal relationship within a society, in which the needs of people with impairments are often given little or no consideration... These barriers prevent them from gaining equal access to information, education, employment, public transport, housing and social/recreational opportunities.'*
> (Carson, 2009 p10)

This understanding has been developed and applied to mental distress, with a shift away from individual symptoms and pathology, towards an understanding that incorporates stigma, discrimination and oppression, as well as recognition of the impact of social situations on mental health issues and how this can contribute to, and prevent, levels of distress.

Within the context of the social model, which continues to be integrated into mental health policy and practice, the impact of the social system and network is of vital importance and can have a significant impact on the individual's recovery. Recovery as an approach is considered in detail in section 5, however, for this competence it must be recognised that the social support system and the response of the individual's network needs to be considered. The role of carers, family, friends, and other social contacts is varied. However, the contribution that these networks make to the individual's recovery is widespread and the involvement and engagement of supporters should be part of all support processes. Personalisation recognises that an individual exists within a social context and consideration of all of these roles and contexts is an important element of assessment and planning.

Case study exercise

Simon is a 25-year-old man who lives with his brother. He was diagnosed with bipolar disorder three years ago and has had some periods of extreme distress throughout this time, including one admission, approximately a year ago, under section 2 of the Mental Health Act (1983) for assessment. He sees a social worker from the community team on a regular basis and also attends a social club at his local MIND centre each week.

At the moment, Simon reports that he is feeling well and would like to see less of his social worker but is concerned that if he is discharged from the team he won't get support when he needs it. Simon's brother takes care of the household jobs such as paying the bills and making sure there is food in the house and Simon pays him board and lodging each week from his benefits. He reports that he finds this comforting as he knows that everything is taken care of, but is also frustrated as he feels that he would not cope if he had to do it himself.

Simon's parents live locally and he sees his mother every day. She is quite worried about him and likes to keep a check on him to make sure he is OK. Simon's father feels that he is an adult now and should be left to get on with his life; this is a source of tension between them. He also has a small group of friends and undertakes voluntary work at a local animal shelter, which was arranged for him by one of his friends. He describes his relationship with colleagues as generally supportive and friendly.

Simon would like to have more independence, saying that although he appreciates his family's support when he is feeling down he would like to try and manage his own life.

- Who has a role to play in Simon's recovery within this situation?

- What is the impact of these relationships on Simon's well-being?

- What are the possible options available to support Simon within a personalised approach, in working towards his goals?

Social capital is one area that has been identified as a key element of the personalised approach. Social capital refers to the social relationships and networks that exist within communities, and there is some evidence that shows that health improvements can be seen in areas where there is strong social capital (De Silva *et al*, 2005; Putnam, 1993; 1995). In the context of a social model of understanding mental distress, social capital includes:

> *'...social relationships, social support, formal and informal social networks, group membership, shared norms, trust, reciprocity and community and civic engagement.'* (Duggan *et al*, 2002, p14)

These relationships and resources help to promote an individual's independence as they are based on reciprocity and partnership between the individual and their community (McKenzie *et al*, 2002), which means that while the person can access social support and be involved in local activities, they also have the opportunity to give back to the community and contribute to their local situation.

It should also be noted that as the social network has an impact on the person's well-being, the person also has an impact on those within their social network. Carers, families, friends and communities have a significant role to play and also have their own needs and aspirations that need to be considered. The emphasis on the informal caring role in government policy includes a National Carer's Strategy, and there is a role for services to play in supporting carers and the wider network to ensure that social capital is supported and maintained.

Competence 3

The ability to respond to the needs of people in an ethical, honest, non-judgemental manner.

Non-judgemental practice is a term that is often used within mental health services and generally refers to an approach that accepts the person as an individual and does not make judgements on their choices and preferences. In order to approach situations in this way the individual needs to be aware of their own values and beliefs and how these impact upon the decisions and actions that they may make.

Recovery and personalisation both concentrate on the individual's needs and strengths, and based on values that emphasise the person's choices and preferences. However, there remains a significant amount of stigma and negative attitudes about mental health issues, which can have an impact on a person's well-being (see section 4 for detailed consideration of the impact of stigma and prejudice). These attitudes can create barriers for individuals in terms of community involvement and social inclusion, both areas which are essential within the personalisation approach and which can affect the ability of services and workers to respond in a non-judgemental way. Everyone sees things in a slightly different way and these differences shape how a person responds to a particular need or issue.

Reflection point

How do your attitudes affect how you respond in situations?

Values-based practice recognises and responds to the diverse needs of individuals (Ray *et al*, 2008) by emphasising that each individual has different roles, strengths, needs and perspectives and support needs to reflect these and ensure that the person remains in control of their situation. The principles that guide this approach include the free will of the individual, seeing the most important part of a person's life as their own view of it, a focus on strengths and being encouraging of personal growth.

Diversity within mental health is an important factor. It can directly contribute to both recovery and well-being and there is a need to ensure that the support provided is responsive to the cultural identities that individuals may have. This can include areas such as race, religion, sexuality and disability, but must also consider family and other social roles, which the individual may undertake. These types of issues can have a huge impact on the individual's well-being and will be considered in more detail in sections 4 and 5.

Competence 4

The ability to encourage active choices and participation in care and treatment.

The personalised approach is focused on choice and control by the service user with the aim of achieving the greatest possible degree of self-determination in life. The choices available will vary according to local area and these will continue to be developed as personal budgets and direct payments are used to purchase new support options for individuals. There is a range of services and support from informal support from the person's social support network to small organisations, user-led services and community groups as well as more traditional service providers and large charitable organisations. The wishes and aspirations of the individual need to inform their choices and contribute to their recovery.

Reflection points

- What options are available in your local area in terms of services, groups, and activities that could contribute to a person's recovery or support their families and carers?
- How do you make sure that a person is aware of all their options and supported to make informed choices?

Involvement and participation in support is an area that has received a lot of attention, with clear benefits being shown from co-production and user-led support (Needham & Carr, 2009). This is reflected in the current government strategy for mental health, which states that involvement is essential to the process of service development and delivery, with one of the actions being:

> *'...ongoing involvement and work with people who use services, their carers, families and communities to develop solutions to improve services and well-being.'*
> (DH, 2009a, p71)

What involvement and participation means can range from involvement in individual decision-making and support planning, to participation in service and strategy planning and development. On an individual level, in order to promote user choice and control there needs to be a partnership between the person and the support services they receive, with involvement in the assessment, planning and delivery of support plans. The person themself is the expert in their own situations, and while professional views can help to inform what might work or what options are available to the individual, this should not be at the expense of the individual's preferences and aspirations. Shared ownership of support and risk management (see section 9 for further discussion on risk) has a range of benefits (Langan & Lindow, 2004), and this can directly contribute to the person's recovery by placing them central to the process and assisting them to control their own situation.

Research has been undertaken that suggests that co-production and participation has significant benefits in terms of both individual outcomes, user satisfaction levels, and the quality of services being delivered (Needham & Carr, 2009; Skidmore *et al*, 2006). The recovery approach also emphasises the role of involvement and participation, recognising that the more empowered the users of services are the more responsive the service. Approaches such as peer support and the direct employment of individuals who have experienced mental health issues within services are some of the ways in which individuals are able to get involved and influence service delivery.

Personalisation emphasises participation at all levels, and there is a need for support providers to involve and include service users and carers and to establish a system of proper accountability to the consumers of services. This level of co-production is something that the mental health sector has historically struggled to achieve, with attitudes and actions being taken by services without full collaboration with the people who changes will most affect. For personalisation to be successful in mental health this must be addressed and workers and services need to be proactive, with representation of users and carers being further developed and more inclusive than is currently the case.

> *'[Putting People First] seeks to be the first public service reform programme which is co-produced, co-developed, co-evaluated and recognises that real change will only be achieved through the participation of users and carers at every stage.'* (DH, 2007, p1)

Competence 5

The ability to conduct a legal, ethical and accountable practice that remains open to the scrutiny of peers and colleagues.

Unlike other areas of health and social care, the use of the Mental Health Act to treat people against their wishes is a factor that needs to be considered within mental health. Everyone within the mental health field needs to be aware of this legislation, and will need to work within it, whether undertaking a specific role or supporting a person who is subject to restrictions as a result of a section of the act.

The Mental Health Act may be put into action when a person's health and safety, or the safety of others is compromised. When intervention is required, which the person is unwilling or unable to agree to, this can make the power relationships that exist within mental health particularly complicated. Being subject to mental health law does not mean that a person does not have rights, and the task of those involved is to make sure that interventions are both legal and ethical and uphold the rights of the individual. The HRA framework provides a basis of rights, which include privacy, dignity and freedom of choice in a number of areas. Services need to make sure that even when liberty may be restricted, this is for a specific purpose and is the least restrictive option available in the circumstances.

Involvement of both the individual and their support network, including family and carers, is needed within this framework to assist with the decisions made, and there is a requirement on professionals to be specific and transparent in the decisions they make. Challenges can be brought and the right to appeal for restrictions is available, to ensure that people are able to make these challenges there is a need to be clear about why decisions have been made and to make all efforts to involve people in the decision making process. Mental health law was changed in November 2008 by the Mental Health Act (2007), which amended the 1983 legislation and introduced a set of guiding principles on which any legal intervention needs to be based. These principles are as follows.

- Purpose principle: decisions are taken to minimise the negative effects of mental health issues and maximise safety, well-being and recovery.
- Least restriction principle: any actions taken without the individual's consent are kept to the minimum necessary.
- Respect principle: actions taken recognise diverse needs, cultures and values, and consider the wishes, feelings and views of the person.
- Participation principle: individuals are involved in planning, developing and reviewing their own support, including the involvement of their carers and family.
- Effectiveness, efficiency and equity principle: the resources available are used to the best available effect, and are applied in an equitable way to meet the individual's needs (DH, 2008, p5–6).

These principles are the framework for ensuring that any support that is provided, which may be against the individual's wishes, considers the individual's rights and preferences.

Accountable practice means that the decisions and actions that are taken are open to scrutiny and challenge. Within the personalised approach this is not just about the scrutiny of peers and colleagues but more importantly service users and carers. For individuals to be able to exercise choice and control there needs to be openness about what is available and why actions are being taken. Involvement in these situations is vital, and the individual's wishes should be considered in any decision-making process.

Case study exercise

Aarif is a 68-year-old man of Indian origin. He has been in England since he was 10 years old when his family emigrated. He has had contact with mental health services for approximately 35 years and has a diagnosis of paranoid schizophrenia. He has two sons who are working in India and one daughter who lives 130 miles away from him. His wife died three months ago and following the funeral his children returned to their respective homes and work. This has left Aarif living alone. He has the support of a social worker from the local community mental health team, and a support worker from a local organisation, which he purchases via a direct payment. He has recently become more distressed and has been offered an informal admission to hospital for assessment and medication review but this could only be offered on an elderly ward where a lot of the patients have dementia. Aarif declined this and has been trying to manage in the community

- How do the principles impact upon Aarif's situation?

- How would you demonstrate these principles in decisions made to promote Aarif's choice and control?

Competence 6

The ability to promote service users' (and carers') rights and responsibilities and recognise and maintain their rights to privacy, dignity, safety, effective treatment and care based on the principle of informed consent.

One of the key roles, for those working within mental health settings, is to ensure that individuals' rights are observed, and this in emphasised within personalisation. The focus on choice and control means that the person has rights to choice and control, and this includes personal dignity and privacy.

A number of studies have tried to define what is meant by dignity in social care settings (Jacelon *et al*, 2004; Bayer *et al*, 2005; Griffin-Heslin, 2005; Woolhead *et al*, 2004), and a number of themes have been highlighted, these include respect, autonomy, empowerment and communication. The SCIE guide *Dignity in Care* (Cass *et al*, 2009), sets out some elements that are needed to promote individual privacy, these are:

- modesty and privacy in personal care
- confidentiality of treatment and personal information
- privacy of personal space (p114).

These things form the basis of an individual's rights to personal dignity within mental health support, and there needs to be an understanding and consideration of how these aspects can impact upon the person's well-being and recovery.

Reflection points

- How do you feel when your privacy is not being considered?
- What impact does this have on your well-being?

Informed consent is a term that means that an individual's decisions are made using the full information available, considering options and being aware of the consequences of the decision. The Department of Health has issued guidance on consent, and states that in order to be valid consent must:

> *'...be given voluntarily by an appropriately informed person who has the capacity to consent to the intervention in question.'* (DH, 2009b, p9)

To be able to give informed consent the person needs to have capacity to make the given decision, the Mental Capacity Act (2005) and its code of practice (DCA, 2007), sets out what capacity means, and states that a person should be presumed to have capacity unless there is evidence to suggest otherwise. This is based on a decision specific and time specific basis. The definition of capacity includes the following.

- The person needs to understand the information relevant to the decision.
- The person can retain the information.
- The person can use and weigh the information to make the decision.
- The person is able to communicate the decision by any means.

It should be noted that just because a person does not have capacity to make one decision it does not necessarily mean they are unable to make another, and each issue needs to be considered separately.

From a personalisation perspective the person's needs and wishes are the central consideration, and this includes informed consent and being able to make decisions about their own lives, including the support they may need to manage mental health issues and promote recovery. Treatment options are varied and the person has a number of choices about how and who provides the support they need.

Competence 7

The ability to work as a member of the therapeutic team in making a safe and effective contribution to the de-escalation and management of anger and violence especially through the use of control and restraint techniques.

There remains an emphasis on the management of violence and aggression as part of the risk management procedures within mental health (see section 9), which recognises that there are times when control and restraint may be needed. While this is a reality of mental health service delivery, it is not as common as the media reports, and mental health practitioners should only use these techniques as a last resort (DH, 2008). The Mental Health Act code of practice (DH, 2008) provides guidance for the use of restraint and this is based on the principles discussed in competence 5 of this section.

Work by the Mental Health Act Commission and the Department of Health have highlighted that there is unequal use of seclusion and restraint processes, with African-Caribbean men in particular, being more likely to undergo formal detention, control, restraint and seclusion within mental health settings (DH, 2005; MHAC, 2006; 2009), and the impact of worker prejudice and wider stigma are suggested to be a factor in this situation (Mental Health Alliance, 2007; MHAC, 2005; Vige, 2005). This emphasises the need for individuals to remain aware of, and address their own values and beliefs within any support or treatment situation. An awareness of cultural responses is also needed as behavioural norms may be misunderstood and can lead to unnecessary intervention. To ensure that the individual's rights and wishes are promoted, there is a need to develop both cultural competence and reflective practice to ensure that decisions are made on an informed basis and not unduly influenced by prejudice and presumptions.

Reflection point

What factors would influence your decisions about whether control and restraint should be used?

De-escalation as a technique involves verbal reassurance, a calm approach and providing time-out facilities, along with others, and these should always be applied as the best option. Training of staff and carers is one way that has been recommended as a means of improving de-escalation, and the involvement of individuals throughout should be a factor that is considered as best practice. Methods such as crisis and contingency planning can be used to apply risk management to these situations and retain the emphasis that the person themself is the expert in what works for them, with a view to avoidance of unnecessary control being placed on a person.

Competence 8

Adherence to local and professionally prescribed codes of ethical conduct and practice.

Different professions and organisations have their own codes of practice, however, these have common themes that need to be in place to make sure support that is provided is ethical and tailored to the individual's needs. The principles of the Mental Health Act code of practice (DH, 2008) provides a strong foundation for any support that is accessed by individuals, and the emphasis on personal choice and control should remain a central consideration regardless of the legal status of the individual.

The common themes that are evident with the codes of conduct and practice in mental health are reflected throughout this workbook, with the essential shared capabilities providing the range of competencies and values-based practice that should be in place for individuals who may need support from services. These are further supported by social care codes of practice and the principles of the personalised approach. The basic principles of personalisation include:

- finding new collaborative ways of working and developing local partnerships, which produce a range of services for people to choose from and opportunities for social inclusion
- tailoring support to people's individual needs – an equality and diversity based approach
- recognising and supporting carers in their role, while enabling them to maintain a life beyond their caring responsibilities

- a total system response so that universal and community services and resources are accessible to everyone
- early intervention and prevention so that people are supported early on and in a way that's right for them (Carr, 2010).

These principles are largely consistent with professional approaches, and emphasise the individual's rights, responsibilities and choices as the central elements of any support that is provided. There is, however, a shift in the power relationship between service and service users, and an increased emphasis on the carer role, which needs to be considered within the practice environment, with the individual leading the process rather than being viewed as a passive recipient of services.

Reflection points

- How do you make sure that a person leads the support planning process?
- What might enable family members and other people who provide support to an individual to be engaged as fully as that individual wishes in their support planning?

Competence 9

Knowledge of policies, practices and procedures concerning the local implementation of mental health and related legislation.

There is a range of policies, practices and procedures that guide the implementation of mental health law and individuals need to ensure that they are aware of their local policies and procedures within their organisations and services. These are based upon national guidance, which is largely delivered in the form of codes of practice. The key guidance that individuals need to familiarise themselves with in terms of the legal frameworks are:

- Mental Health Act Code of Practice – Available online at: http://www.dh.gov.uk/prod_consum_dh/groups/dh_digitalassets/@dh/@en/documents/digitalasset/dh_087073.pdf
- Mental Capacity Act Code of Practice – Available online at: http://www.dca.gov.uk/legal-policy/mental-capacity/mca-cp.pdf
- Deprivation of Liberty Safeguards Code of Practice – Available online at: http://www.dh.gov.uk/prod_consum_dh/groups/dh_digitalassets/@dh/@en/documents/digitalasset/dh_087309.pdf

These codes provide guidance on best practice within the legal frameworks and are all based upon principles that emphasise individual rights as provided by the Human Rights Act. While there are circumstances that may need restrictions to be placed on individuals, this does not mean that these cannot be carried out within a person-centred environment, and involvement of the individual and their carer/families should be a key element of any intervention. Choice and control can be difficult to achieve in circumstances where legal restrictions are in place, however, individuals are still able to make choices about their support and treatment and should be assisted to participate as much as possible, with their wishes and preferences informing what action is taken.

Reflection points

- How do you make sure that an individual's wishes are considered in the process of applying legal restrictions?
- What choices and control can an individual exercise within the legal framework?

Competence 10

The ability to work within the boundaries of local complaints management systems.

Anyone who accesses support providers has the right to make a complaint if they feel they have not received the service they should have, or if they have been treated unfairly or are otherwise dissatisfied with the support they have received. Each organisation has its own complaints system and the individual has a right to access this system. Complaints and feedback should be treated as a learning opportunity for services, incorporating views into service delivery to improve the individual experiences of service users. Complaints are a means by which individuals can provide feedback and directly influence the way services are developed and delivered, and workers have a responsibility to make sure individuals know how to make a complaint if they wish to do so. From April 2009 a single complaint system for NHS and local authority services was introduced, this is based on six key principles, which focus on customer care and respond to the concerns of those who access services. These principles are:

- getting it right
- being customer focused
- being open and accountable
- acting fairly and proportionately
- putting things right
- seeking continuous improvement (DH, 2009a).

Guidance has been published by the Department of Health (DH, 2009a), which sets out what a person can expect, and the principles of a personal approach are included within this, stating as a key aim, that people who use services, regardless of their needs or background should find it easier to make a complaint or provide feedback on the services they access.

Reflection point

How do you make a complaint within your organisational context?

There is a range of advocacy services available to individuals to support them to make complaints if they need to. In the case of NHS services there is a specific agency that can assist, known as the independent complaints advocacy service (ICAS). For other services, general and other specific advocacy agencies will support the person to make the complaint.

Reflection point

What are the advocacy services in your area that can provide support to a person making a complaint about a mental health support service?

Summary

Section 3 has considered the ethical and legal frameworks in which mental health support operates, and specifically has considered the following capability.

Recognising the rights and aspirations of service users and their families, acknowledging power differentials and minimising them whenever possible. Providing treatment and care that is accountable to service users and carers within the boundaries prescribed by national (professional), legal and local codes of ethical practice.

Legal frameworks can have the effect of both promoting and restricting an individual's rights and liberties, and there are circumstances where an individual's health and safety is at such a risk that they may need treatment against their wishes. In these circumstances, involvement and participation must be encouraged and only the least amount of restriction necessary should be applied. Personalisation supports choice and control and this capability has considered how this can be put into place when some elements of a person's choices are restricted.

Summary exercise

Write a short summary of what this capability means to you in your context/practice, and then answer the following three questions.

- What have you learnt by completing this section?

- How have you now reached competence in this area?

- What do you need to do to maintain your competence?

References

Bayer T, Tadd W & Krajcik S (2005) Dignity: the voice of older people. *Quality in Ageing: Policy, practice and research* **6** 22–29.

Beresford P (2002) Thinking about 'mental health': towards a social model. *Journal of Mental Health* **11** (6) 581–584.

Bloch S & Green SA (2006) An ethical framework for psychiatry. *British Journal of Psychiatry* **188** 7–12.

Bogg D (2008) *The Integration of Mental Health Social Work and the NHS*. Exeter: Learning Matters.

Carson G (2009) *The Social Model of Disability*. Glasgow: Scottish Accessible Information Forum/TSO.

Carr S (2010) *Personalisation: A rough guide* (2nd ed). London: SCIE.

Cass E, Robins D & Richardson A (2009) *Dignity in Care: SCIE Guide 15*. London: SCIE.

Department of Constitutional Affairs (DCA) (2007) *Mental Capacity Act 2005 Code of Practice*. London: TSO.

Department of Health (2005) *Delivering Race Equality in Mental Health Care: An action plan for reform inside and outside services and the government's response to the independent inquiry into the death of David Bennett*. London: DH.

Department of Health (2007) *Putting People First: Transforming adult social care* [online]. London: Department of Health. Available at: http://www.dh.gov.uk/en/Publicationsandstatistics/Publications/PublicationsPolicyAndGuidance/DH_089665 (accessed June 2010).

Department of Health (2008) *Code of Practice: Mental Health Act 1983*. London: TSO.

Department of Health (2009a) *New Horizons: A shared vision for mental health*. London: TSO.

Department of Health (2009b) *Reference Guide to Consent for Examination or Treatment* (2nd ed). London: TSO.

De Silva M, McKenzie K, Harpham T & Huttly SRA (2005) Social capital and mental illness: a systematic review. *Journal of Epidemiology and Community Health* **59** 619–627.

Duggan M with Cooper A & Foster J (2002) *Modernising The Social Model In Mental Health: A discussion paper*. Leeds: Social Perspectives Network/Training Organisation for Personal Social Services (England) (TOPSS).

Griffin-Heslin VL (2005) An analysis of the concept dignity. *Accident and Emergency Nursing* **13** 251–257.

Jacelon CS, Connelly TW, Brown R, Proulx K & Vo T (2004) A concept analysis of dignity for older adults. *Journal of Advanced Nursing* **48** 76–83.

Langan J & Lindow V (2004) *Living with Risk: Mental health service user involvement in risk assessment and management*. Bristol: Policy Press.

Macdonald JE & Beck-Dudley CL (1994) Are deontology and teleology mutually exclusive? *Journal of Business Ethics* **13** (8) 615–623.

McKenzie K, Whitely R & Weich S (2002) Social Capital and Mental Health. *British Journal of Psychiatry* **181** 280–283.

Mental Health Alliance (2007) *Black and Minority Ethnic Mental Health Service Users*. Briefing for the second reading of the mental health bill in the House of Lords [online]. Available at: http://www.mentalhealthalliance.org.uk/policy/documents/BME_Briefing_2nd_Reading.pdf (accessed June 2010).

MHAC (2005) *Count Me In: The national mental health and ethnicity census. 2005 service user survey*. London: TSO.

MHAC (2006) *In Place of Fear? Eleventh biennial report 2003–2005*. London: TSO.

MHAC (2009) *Coercion and Consent. Thirteenth biennial report 2007–2009*. London: TSO.

Needham C & Carr S (2009) *Co-production: An emerging evidence base for adult social care transformation.* Research Briefing 31 [online]. London: SCIE. Available at: http://www.scie.org.uk/publications/briefings/files/briefing31.pdf (accessed June 2010).

Putnam RD (1993) *Making Democracy Work: Civic traditions in modern Italy*. Princeton, NJ: Princeton University Press.

Putnam RD (1995) Bowling alone: America's declining social capital. *Journal of Democracy* **1** (6) 65–78.

Ray M, Pugh R, Roberts D & Beech B (2008) Mental Health and Social Work. *Research Briefing* **26**. London: SCIE.

Skidmore P, Bound K. & Lownsbrough H (2006) *Community Participation: Who benefits?* York: Joseph Rowntree Foundation.

Tew J, Beresford P, Plumb S, Ferns P, Wallcraft J, Williams J & Carr S (2002) *Start Making Sense. Developing social models to understand and work with mental distress.* SPN study day 11 November 2002. London: SPN/SCIE.

Vige M (2005) Race and mental health treatment. *Criminal Justice Matters* **61** (1) 28–30.

Woolhead G, Calnan M, Dieppe P & Tadd W (2004) Dignity in older age – what do older people in the United Kingdom think? *Age and Ageing* **33** 165–169.

Section 4: Challenging inequality

Addressing the causes and consequences of stigma, discrimination, social inequality and exclusion on service users, carers and mental health services. Creating, developing or maintaining valued social roles for people in the communities they come from.

A great deal of attention has been placed on the impact of the social system on an individual's well-being, and it has been demonstrated that the individual's inclusion in their local communities can have a direct connection to their recovery from a mental health problem (DH, 2009a; Sayce, 2001; Huxley & Thornicroft, 2003; RCP, 2009; NSIP, 2009). As such, the existence of inequality and stigma within society towards those experiencing mental distress is something that needs to be challenged and addressed wherever possible.

The personalisation agenda includes the role of social capital as a core element of the approach, and as such, this competence is a key area for practitioners who are delivering a personalised approach to mental health care.

Aims

This section of the workbook will assist workers, service users and carers to consider the impact of discrimination and stigma and the ways it can be challenged in day-to-day practice. The overall aims of this section are:

- to understand the role of social capital within mental health care
- to develop an understanding of the impact of discrimination, exclusion, inequality and stigma, on an individual's recovery
- to consider strategies that can be developed to address and challenge discrimination.

Overview

The understanding of the role and impact of discrimination and stigma is well developed within the mental health field. The social aspects of an individual's life can have a significant influence on their personal recovery, and as a result social inclusion principles are now central to mental health strategy and service development.

There are seven areas of competence in this shared capability, these are:

Competence 1:	Understand the nature of stigma.
Competence 2:	Understand the effects of exclusion and discrimination.
Competence 3:	Understand the role that mental health services play in creating and maintaining inequality and discrimination.
Competence 4:	Understand the role that services have to play in fighting inequality and discrimination.
Competence 5:	Demonstrate the ability to challenge inequality and discrimination within their role.
Competence 6:	Demonstrate the ability to communicate their concerns to others within the care system.
Competence 7:	Demonstrate the ability to know when there is little more they can do and recognise the limits of their competence.

Significant research has been carried out in the area of social exclusion and stigma and it is useful to have an awareness of the evidence base. This will assist the reader to understand the context in which discrimination and stigma occurs and the impact it can have on individuals and groups.

By working through this section readers will be able to link inequality and social inclusion issues to their day-to-day experience of delivering or receiving mental health services, and understand the impact of the social aspects of an individual's experience.

Competence 1

Understand the nature of stigma.

The definition of stigma is '*a mark or sign of disgrace or discredit*' (Oxford English Dictionary) and it can be seen as a negative attitude, usually based on ignorance, prejudice and fear, towards a particular person, group or issue. In general terms it refers to the negative effects experienced by a group or an individual as a result of the attitudes in society, for example, certain age groups, religions, or racial groups have an association or stereotype attached to them which means that people who appear to be from that group will be treated in a certain way (Haywood & Bright, 1997; Corrigan & Matthews, 2003; Link & Phelan, 2001).

In the case of people with mental health difficulties this stigma is often based on fear of dangerousness, a presumed lack of capacity or the inability to care for or protect themselves (Thornicroft, 2006; Beresford, 2005; Byrne, 2000), and as a result society's response is to either avoid, exclude or apply significant restrictions on the individual. This response is often not based on individual behaviour, but rather the presumptions that exist about how someone with the label of mental illness will behave.

Reflective exercise

Consider the terms listed, and answer the following questions:

Teenager	Injecting drug user	Binge drinker
Gay man	Single mother	Christian
Schizophrenic	Grandparent	Art teacher

- What thoughts, images or ideas come to mind when you think about these terms?

- Where do these thoughts or ideas come from? What are they based on?

- How do these thoughts, images or ideas affect how you behave towards someone with one of these labels?

There are different types of stigma, and a great deal of research has been carried out, both within the general sociological themes of the social role of stigma, and also with specific relevance to mental health issues.

Stigma can arise as a result of an actual or perceived difference. The work of Goffman (1963), which was an important development within sociological thought on the subject, stated that there were three types of stigma. These were stigma as a result of physical differences, perceived character and behavioural differences, or social differences, such as association or belonging to a particular group. In terms of mental health, the last two areas are particularly relevant – the stereotypes that exist within society about someone with a mental health problem are largely related to perceived ideas such as those presented by the media rather than based on the reality of what having mental health issues mean, and these assumptions can lead to exclusion and discriminatory attitudes towards those it affects. In addition to stigma from others a further type of stigma has been identified – self-stigma (Kanter *et al*, 2008; Corrigan & Watson, 2006; Byrne, 2000). It appears that those who experience mental health difficulties apply the same labels to themselves as the rest of society and this can lead to feelings of guilt and shame and withdrawal from social interaction.

Public attitudes towards mental health issues have been studied on a regular basis by the Department of Health since 1994 (DH, 2000; 2003; 2007a; 2008; 2009a). These surveys ask members of the public a number of questions regarding their views of mental health problems and people who experience them. Both positive and negative opinions are included, and participants are asked to agree or disagree with a range of statements. Two examples of these statements are '*people with mental health problems are less dangerous than most people think*' and '*people with mental health problems are incapable of making simple decisions*' with participants asked to state whether they agree or disagree. While the survey shows that there has been a decrease in negative attitudes overall, there is still 39% of participants who believe that people with mental health problems are dangerous and 32% who believe they are unable to make decisions. The persistence of discriminatory attitudes and stigma was further demonstrated in a survey undertaken by Time to Change in 2008, the project – *Stigma shout* – surveyed over 3,000 people and found that 87% of participants had experienced discrimination as a result of their mental health problems and 71% reported that it prevented them from doing the things they wanted to do.

It is clear that discrimination and stigma exist within society and amongst individuals for a variety of reasons, and these are based on ignorance of the subject, which leads to prejudices and stereotypes being formed. In the case of mental health problems there is a range of negative beliefs that are evident, and these are embedded in social thinking and supported by media images. These attitudes represent a challenge to the personalisation agenda as social capital and universal services both rest on the principle of inclusion and community engagement, areas that in mental health can be directly affected by negative stereotypes and stigma.

Competence 2

Understand the effects of exclusion and discrimination.

It is clear that discrimination and stigma towards people with mental health problems is widespread within society, and while these attitudes have improved over time there is still a significant proportion of people who experience exclusion and stigma as a result of their mental health difficulties. The effects of these attitudes are widespread and in order to challenge such prejudices it is helpful to be aware of the full range of influences stigma can have on an individual's recovery and overall quality of life.

Some of the key impacts of discrimination are set out in the aims of the Time to Change campaign, which is a current England UK-wide programme, run by MIND and Rethink, aimed at ending the discrimination faced by people with mental health problems, these are stigma that can:

- isolate people
- exclude people from day-to-day activities
- stop people getting and keeping jobs
- prevent people seeking help
- have a negative impact on physical health
- delay treatment and impair recovery (see www.time-to-change.org.uk).

As will be presented in section 5 of this workbook, an individual's recovery is based on a number of elements, including social interaction, help-seeking, and meaningful activity, and if societal attitudes prevent people from accessing and engaging in these areas then exclusion, discrimination and stigma may represent a significant barrier to an individual's recovery.

Case study exercise

Sarah is a 29-year-old single woman. She is from a large family and has three brothers and one sister all of who live in the local area. Sarah has a daughter, who is now 10 years old, and who lives with her grandparents.

Sarah left school at 16 and has three GSCEs. She started a diploma course at her local college in business and administration when she was 23 but did not complete the course. She went back to college last year and now has her diploma. She has worked on and off over the last few years, mainly in shop work or temporary secretary positions. Her last job was 18 months ago prior to restarting her college course.

After leaving school Sarah spent a lot of her time with a group who were known for antisocial behaviour around town, with a reputation for drinking and taking drugs and regular visits from local police. Sarah was pregnant at 19 and her parents suggested that she and her new daughter should live with them. She found it difficult living with her parents, and her behaviour became increasingly chaotic. She often went 'missing' for several days at a time; she drank heavily and used a range of drugs recreationally. Sarah was arrested for possession of cannabis and shop theft and given a two-year probation order when she was 20 years old. She completed the order and has not offended since. During this period of her life Sarah found it difficult to cope. She became very isolated and her relationship with her mother became strained. Following an argument Sarah became very distressed and took an overdose. She was admitted to the local hospital and was seen by the duty psychiatrist who referred her to the community mental health team for assessment. She was seen by a community psychiatric nurse for about six months and was then discharged from the service. She has not needed service support since then, but has seen her GP and was prescribed a short course of antidepressants following a family bereavement.

Sarah is now applying for jobs after receiving her diploma in business and administration, and is concerned about disclosing her history on her applications.

- From the information provided, identify the areas in Sarah's case that may be subject to stigma or discrimination.

There is a substantial body of research into the areas of social inclusion (SEU, 2003; NSIP, 2009; Huxley & Thornicroft, 2003) and the impact of stigma on mental health (Cass *et al*, 2009; Time to Change, 2009; Byrne, 2000; DH, 2009b), and the evidence is clear that in order to promote independence and quality of life, community inclusion is required. This is reflected in the national mental health strategy *New Horizons* (DH, 2009a), which places aspects such as equality, employment, housing, and community support, as the central focus for the next 10 years of service delivery. The personalisation of mental health care is also a key element of the strategy, and it states that '*personalised care is fundamental to a recovery approach*' (p29). In order to achieve personalisation, negative attitudes to mental health problems must be addressed. The elements of developing social capital and the role of universal services are both areas in which discrimination and stigma can be barriers to the personalised approach. Using universal services as an example – primary care has a significant role to play and the promotion of physical health services for individuals who also have a mental health problem.

Yet according to figures from Rethink, people with schizophrenia and bipolar disorder are at a higher than average risk of a range of conditions, including cardiovascular and respiratory diseases (Rethink, 2006). There is a range of explanations for these rates, including access to good primary health services, presumptions made by professionals about the concerns of an individual with mental health problems, a higher likelihood of unhealthy or risky lifestyle choices and higher rates of deprivation and poverty, all of which can contribute to both the health inequalities and the responses from universal service providers.

The same types of issues can be seen in other sectors such as relationships, housing and employment, all of which are also significant within the personalisation agenda. For example, a recent survey has shown that 92% of people believe that admitting to having a mental health problem would damage their career (Time to Change, 2009). This type of view has not changed significantly over time. A MIND survey in 2004 showed that 84% of people experienced problems getting jobs, mortgages and relationships, and an earlier study (Read & Baker, 1996) showed that 34% of people with mental health problems reported that they had been dismissed or forced to resign from a job.

Education, information and support for mainstream services and the wider community, to assist in understanding the needs of individuals with mental health problems is one way in which discrimination can be challenged, and both service users and workers have a role to play in delivering this.

Practice examples

Education not discrimination (END)

Part of the Time for Change project, END targets key audiences who have a significant impact on the lives of people with mental health problems. The aim of the project is to carry out practical work with specific groups of people and make a positive difference to their knowledge, attitudes and behaviour towards mental health.

The target groups are:

- four medical schools (3,112 students over four years)
- four teacher training universities/colleges (720 students over four years)
- trainee head teachers
- social inclusion officers (pastoral care leads in schools).

Action on stigma programme

The programme is part of the SHIFT stigma campaign, and is for people with an interest in reducing the stigma and discrimination directed towards people in the workplace. Shift has published the *Line Manager's Resource*, a booklet and website that gives advice and information for managing and supporting people with mental health problems in the workplace. The resource also gives advice and information for employees to help them assess their own needs and plan for meetings with their manager.

Employment project: eastern region

Employment workers set up a series of 'business breakfasts' with local businesses and chamber of commerce representatives. The focus of these meetings was to provide information and advice to local employers and provide a forum for employers and individuals with mental health problems to talk to each other in an informal setting. The aim being to provide support to both employers and individuals and break down some of the barriers and attitudes among business people in the local community in order to promote inclusive recruitment practices.

Competence 3

Understand the role that mental health services play in creating and maintaining inequality and discrimination.

The views and values of wider society can also be seen within services and professional groups, and research has shown that professionals can play a key role in stigmatising individuals with mental health problems (Lauber *et al*, 2006; Verhaeghe *et al*, 2007; Nordt *et al*, 2006). Services that are offered to individuals, and the organisations delivering these services, can contribute to the way individuals are viewed, and increase the discrimination and stigmatisation of certain groups.

The role of services in inequality and discrimination is a real issue for the transforming social care agenda, as it presents a range of barriers to realising the vision of personalised services. The take up of direct payments is an example of these barriers for mental health care. Despite the introduction of direct payments in 1997, research carried out from 2000 to 2003 by the Health and Social Care Advisory Service (HASCAS) found that most local authorities had very few individuals in receipt of this service. A number of explanations for this were offered, and these included concerns by professionals about risk, which restricted their willingness to access payments on behalf of service users (Newbigging & Lowe, 2005). A recent study conducted by MIND, which reviewed the evidence for personalisation from a mental health perspective, has shown that in comparison to other groups, mental health direct payments are still a lot lower than for other service user groups (MIND, 2009).

This has been further explored by a number of studies (Spandler & Vick, 2004; Cestari *et al*, 2006; Taylor, 2008), which identified a range of issues that were barriers to self-directed support (in these cases direct payments) for people with mental health difficulties, including:

- eligibility for services for individuals whose conditions change
- the perceived capability of individuals to manage their own care and support
- care co-ordinators acting as gatekeepers and concerns about risk.

These explanations suggest that services and professionals continue to have pre-conceived ideas concerning individuals with mental health difficulties, and with this being the case it is no surprise that society mirrors such views.

Case study exercises

Read the following case examples and identify the areas where attitudes of services are impacting upon the individual's choice and control.

(a) Karen has been a user of her local mental health services for several years as a result of depression and anxiety. She has recently had a review of her care and told her care co-ordinator that she would like to make some changes to her care plan and would like some information about direct payments as she thinks that a personal assistant would be helpful for her to access community activities. Her care co-ordinator and her psychiatrist reviewed the plan and said they were concerned about Karen having a direct payment as they felt her mental health needed to be monitored by professionals and the rest of her care plan needed to stay the same, as she is currently stable.

(b) Darren has a 'dual diagnosis' of personality disorder and substance misuse. About 12 months ago he went into a rehabilitation placement, which he completed successfully and he has been drug-free for six months. Darren is finding it difficult at the moment as he is quite isolated and has not been able to make new friends. He has made contact with a local employment project as he wants to learn some new skills and return to work. The worker at the employment project assessed him last week and said that they would not be able to place him anywhere were money changed hands as a result of his drug history, and also queried whether he was ready to take on proper work, saying that they would need some information from his psychiatrist before taking him onto their permitted work scheme.

Promoting choice and control and positive risk within mental health services is needed to be able to roll out personalised support, with service users taking a more active role in designing their support and being a partner rather than a passive recipient in the process. This is a culture shift for many services, and professional anxieties and misconceptions are barriers that need to be overcome.

While it is recognised that exposure to mental health issues in the general population can reduce stigma (Alexander & Link, 2003), this is not always the case within services, and the perceived and actual attitudes of professionals and services continues to be an issue for individuals with mental health problems.

Competence 4

Understand the role that services have to play in fighting inequality and discrimination.

Although it has been shown that a range of attitudes exist within services that contribute to maintaining the stigmatisation of mental health, it is also the case that services have a significant role to play in helping to break down social discrimination and inequalities. Studies into inequality have shown that individuals with mental health problems are more likely to experience a wide range of health and social issues (McKenzie *et al*, 2002; Murali & Oyebode, 2004; Blank *et al*, 2004; Wildman, 2003), examples include physical health problems, unemployment, poverty and unstable housing. These are all areas in which services can support individuals to challenge and improve their situations, and as such, contribute to the fight against inequality for those with mental health difficulties.

Providing reliable information and engaging with local communities can assist in reducing negative attitudes towards mental health. A large amount of the discrimination that exists is based upon misconception and a lack of information and understanding of what having a mental health problem means. While there are many national campaigns that use social marketing to promote positive images of mental health problems, there remains a need for local services to have a visible presence in the debate/action, both in the health and social care sectors and more widely across public and community services. Additionally, services that link with local businesses, employers, education establishments, and community groups tend to have a wider network on which to draw, and are able to facilitate a greater range of opportunities for the users and carers within their services. To be able to provide a personalised approach, services need to actively play a role in promoting accurate information and links with the full range of services and groups in order to be capable of responding to the diversity of needs that may arise. Social capital is a significant factor in the personalisation agenda, and as such, services need to look beyond the silo of health and social care provision and access wider community involvement options with the users of their services.

Activity

Considering your local area, identify the range of contacts and groups that exist, then those that your service is involved with, and identify any gaps where there is not currently any link.

What can be done to address the gaps identified?

Competence 5

Demonstrate the ability to challenge inequality and discrimination within their role.

Challenging inequality and discrimination within their role is a key competence for all within the mental health system, whether they are professionals or user-led groups and representatives and carers. Being able to develop a wide network of groups and services and provide support to universal services in terms of information and advice is a key part of this, and workers in particular need to be able to identify and challenge inequality as they come across it. As discussed in the previous competencies within this section of the workbook, workers should not accept presumptions about individuals with mental health problems, and they need to be aware that indirect discrimination can be as powerful as direct discrimination and inequality. Issues such as poor access to physical health care, or the reluctance of employers to engage the services of individuals with difficulties are two examples of the types of inequality that may be encountered, and individuals need to be comfortable with pointing out these issues as they are encountered and working towards counteracting the effect of such concerns and anxieties wherever possible.

Everyone has a role to play in addressing the discrimination that individuals face, and this is often carried out on an individual level. Challenging attitudes and cultures can be a daunting task. However, mental health workers have a duty to point out issues as they are encountered in day-to-day practice, and ensure that the rights of individuals are upheld. Under the Disability

Discrimination Act (1995) it is an offence to discriminate against an individual on the basis of a disability, which includes a mental health problem, and individual rights need to be considered at all times. Support services such as advocacy is one of the methods that can be used to ensure that individuals' rights, views and wishes are observed and workers need to be aware of the range of advocacy services that are available in the local area and how these are accessed. Within the personalisation approach, social systems, universal services, and individual choice and control are all aspects that need to be in place, and the stigma of mental illness can be a significant barrier to each of these. Workers need to be confident in their ability to challenge such views and issues and be aware of where support can be accessed to assist them in this task.

Reflection points

- What are some of the areas of inequality that you have encountered in your area?
- How would you challenge negative attitudes when you identify them? Consider what you would say/do if faced with someone refusing access or expressing a negative view about an individual with mental health problems.

Competence 6

Demonstrate the ability to communicate their concerns to others within the care system.

Being able to work and respond to individual needs with creativity and energy is a requirement for those within mental health services. However, this is not something that is carried out independently. Co-operation and communication is needed and when considering personalisation and social inclusion, a whole range of networks and links need to be made in order to ensure the greatest possible range of choices and options for people. From a personalisation perspective this is a crucial competence as a range of services, groups and social supports need to be drawn on to ensure choices are available that are responsive to the diversity. Mental health issues affect one in four of the population, and as such, the needs and aspirations that people have span the full range of social groups, situations and abilities.

Care planning and risk management processes, which are shared activities, need to be a central element of the support system (DH, 2007b; DH, 2007c; Langan & Lindow, 2004; Morgan, 2007a) within both personalisation and recovery approaches. Partnership between individuals and the services they access, which are clear about risks and needs, can help to ensure that the person retains ownership of their own situations while still being able to identify and remain aware of any possible risks. This shared approach is consistent with the ideas of co-production, which are embedded within the personalised approach, and places the control with the user rather than with the professional. In addition, confidentiality is an issue that is often encountered within services, and there is a need for workers to understand local protocols and ensure that individuals using services are aware of the limits to confidentiality and their rights under these arrangements. Advanced statements and information agreements between service users and workers are two of the key ways that the issue of information sharing can be approached. It is important that there is transparency and honesty about what will and will not be shared, and this should form the basis of any working relationship.

Case study exercise

Irena is a 22-year-old woman who has been accessing mental health services since her late teens as a result of periods of self-harm. This has largely taken the form of cutting herself with scissors. Irena has recently undertaken a vocational assessment and she has expressed a desire to train as a hairdresser.

- Identify a shared risk management plan, which would share the risk, and support Irena in her aim.

Competence 7

Demonstrate the ability to know when there is little more they can do and recognise the limits of their competence.

Training and professional development are important factors in the delivery of mental health care – whether as a worker needing to keep up to date with professional registration, or as a service user getting involved with service developments and improvements. Personalisation is a new approach, and stakeholders need to make sure that they have access to information, advice, supervision and training to be able to engage with the developments.

Positive risk taking and the role of personal and individual budgets in promoting choice and control are two of the areas that mental health staff and service users will need to become familiar and comfortable with if personalisation is to become a reality in mental health services. This poses a huge challenge to the mental health system, which also has certain duties of care to both individuals and the wider community, and as such, there is a clear need to implement a culture of managing and minimising risk within services, while still promoting choice and control for users. Positive risk (Morgan, 2004; Morgan, 2007a; Morgan, 2007b) has received a great deal of attention over the past decade and is supported by the policy frameworks, along with shared ownership of risk between individuals and services (DH, 2007b; 2007c). Workers need to ensure that they undertake risk assessments that identify trends, indicators and contexts alongside the individual's (and their significant other's) views. These need to be well documented to evidence how decisions are made, and where possible, agreement with this assessment. However, there also needs to be an acknowledgement that there are still occasions where things will go wrong, and this may be unavoidable rather than a product of a flawed system.

Summary

This section has considered the capability of 'challenging inequality' within mental health and how this applies to the personalisation approach. The definition of this capability within the 10 Essential Shared Capabilities is:

> *'Addressing the causes and consequences of stigma, discrimination, social inequality and exclusion on service users, carers and mental health services. Creating, developing or maintaining valued social roles for people in the communities they come from.'*

These competencies have explored the impact of stigma and discrimination towards individuals with mental health issues, and highlighted some of the impacts that such attitudes can have on individual's recovery, well-being and social interactions. While it is recognised that changing culture and attitudes is a long-term campaign, it is part of the role of all individuals and services within the mental health system to challenge attitudes as they are encountered, and provide support, education and information to help break down some of the barriers that discrimination and stigma can create.

Summary exercise

Write a short summary of what this capability means to you in your context/practice, and then answer the following three questions.

- What have you learnt by completing this section?

- How have you now reached competence in this area?

- What do you need to do to maintain your competence?

References

Alexander L & Link B (2003) The impact of contact on stigmatising attitudes toward people with mental illness. *Journal of Mental Health* **12** (3) 271–289.

Beresford P (2005) Social approaches to madness and distress: user perspectives and user knowledge. In: J Tew (Ed) *Social Perspectives in Mental Health: Developing social models to understand and work with mental distress*. London: Jessica Kingsley Publishers.

Blank L, Ellis L, Goyder E & Peters J (2004) *Tackling Inequalities in Mental Health – The experience of new deal for communities*. Research Report 34. Sheffield: Sheffield Hallam University.

Byrne P (2000) Stigma of mental illness and ways to diminish it. *Advances in Psychiatric Treatment* **6** 65–72.

Cass E, Robbins D & Richardson A (2009) *Dignity in Care within Mental Health: Tackling stigma*. Guide 15. (3rd update). London: SCIE.

Cestari L, Munroe M, Evans S, Smith A & Huxley P (2006) Fair access to care services (FACS): implementation in the mental health context of the UK. *Health and Social Care in the Community* **14** (6) 474–481.

Corrigan PW & Matthews AK (2003) Stigma and disclosure: implications for coming out of the closet. *Journal of Mental Health* **12** (3) 235–270.

Corrigan PW & Watson AC (2006) The paradox of self-stigma and mental illness. *Clinical Psychology: Science and practice* **9** (1) 35–53.

Department of Health (2000) *Attitudes to Mental Illness Research Report 2000* [online]. Available at: http://www.dh.gov.uk/en/Publicationsandstatistics/PublishedSurvey/ListOfSurveySince1990/Surveylistmentalhealth/index.htm (accessed June 2010).

Department of Health (2003) *Attitudes to Mental Illness Research Report 2000* [online]. Available at: http://www.dh.gov.uk/en/Publicationsandstatistics/PublishedSurvey/ListOfSurveySince1990/Surveylistmentalhealth/index.htm (accessed June 2010).

Department of Health (2007a) *Attitudes to Mental Illness Research Report 2000* [online]. Available at: http://www.dh.gov.uk/en/Publicationsandstatistics/PublishedSurvey/ListOfSurveySince1990/Surveylistmentalhealth/index.htm (accessed June 2010).

Department of Health (2007b) *Independence, Choice and Risk: A guide to best practice in supported decision making*. London: TSO.

Department of Health (2007c) *Best Practice in Managing Risk: Principles and evidence for best practice in the assessment and management of risk to self and others in mental health services*. London: TSO.

Department of Health (2008) *Attitudes to Mental Illness Research Report 2000* [online]. Available at: http://www.dh.gov.uk/en/Publicationsandstatistics/PublishedSurvey/ListOfSurveySince1990/Surveylistmentalhealth/index.htm (accessed June 2010).

Department of Health (2009a) *New Horizons: Working together for better mental health*. London: TSO.

Department of Health (2009b) *Attitudes to Mental Illness Research Report 2009* [online]. Available at: http://www.dh.gov.uk/en/Publicationsandstatistics/PublishedSurvey/ListOfSurveySince1990/Surveylistmentalhealth/index.htm (accessed June 2010).

Goffman E (1963) *Stigma: Notes on the management of spoiled identity*. Harlow: Prentice-Hall.

Haywood P & Bright JA (1997) Stigma and Mental Illness: A critique and review. *Journal of Mental Health* **6** (4) 345–354.

Huxley P & Thornicroft G (2003) Social inclusion, social quality and mental illness. *British Journal of Psychiatry* **182** (4) 289–290.

Kanter JW, Rusch LC & Brondino MJ (2008) Depression self-stigma: a new measure and preliminary findings. *Journal of Nervous and Mental Diseases* **196** (9) 663–670.

Langan J & Lindow V (2004) *Living with Risk: Mental health service user involvement in risk assessment and management*. Bristol: Polity Press/Joseph Rowntree Foundation.

Lauber C, Nordt C, Braunschweig C & Rossler W (2006) Do mental health professionals stigmatise their patients? *Acta Psychiatrica Scandinavica* **113** (s429) 51–59.

Link B & Phelan J (2001) Conceptualising stigma. *Annual Review of Sociology* **27** (1) 363–385.

McKenzie K, Whitely R & Weich S (2002) Social capital and mental health. *British Journal of Psychiatry* **181** 280-283.

MIND (2009) *Personalisation in Mental Health: A review of the evidence* [online]. London: MIND. Available at: http://www.mind.org.uk/assets/0000/2164/putting_us_first_personalisation.pdf (accessed June 2010).

Morgan S (2004) Positive risk-taking: an idea whose time has come. *Health Care Risk Report*, October 18–19.

Morgan S (2007a) Working with risk. *Mental Health Today* 36–37.

Morgan S (2007b) *Working with Risk Practitioner's Manual*. Brighton: Pavilion Publishing.

Murali V & Oyebode F (2004) Poverty, Social inequality and mental health. *Advances in Psychiartric Treatment* **10** 216–224.

National Social Inclusion Programme (2009) *Vision and Progress: Social inclusion and mental health* [online]. London: NSIP. Available at: http://www.socialinclusion.org.uk/publications/NSIP_Vision_and_Progress.pdf (accessed June 2010).

Newbigging K & Lowe J (2005) *Implementing Direct Payments in Mental Health*. York: Joseph Rowntree Foundation.

Nordt C, Rossler W & Lauber C (2006) Attitudes of mental health professionals towards people with schizophrenia and major depression. *Schizophrenia Bulletin* **32** (4) 709–714.

Oxford English Dictionary (2008) (11th Edition) Oxford: Oxford University Press.

Read J & Baker S (1996) *Not Just Sticks and Stones: A survey of the stigma, taboos and discrimination experienced by people with mental health problems* [online]. London: Mind.

Available at: http://www.leeds.ac.uk/disability-studies/archiveuk/MIND/MIND.pdf (accessed June 2010).

Rethink (2006) *Briefing – Physical Health and Mental Health* [online]. Available at: http://www.rethink.org/how_we_can_help/news_and_media/briefing_notes/briefing_5.html (accessed June 2010).

Royal College of Psychiatrists Social Inclusion Scoping Group (2009) *Mental Health and Social Inclusion: Position statement* [online]. Available at: http://www.rcpsych.ac.uk/pdf/social%20inclusion%20position%20statement09.pdf (accessed June 2010).

Sayce L (2001) Social inclusion and mental health. *Psychiatric Bulletin* **25** 121–123.

Social Exclusion Unit (2003) *Mental Health and Social Exclusion*. TSO: London.

Spandler H & Vick N (2004) *Direct Payments, Independent Living and Mental Health* [online]. London: Health and Social Care Advisory Service. Available at: www.hascas.org.uk/pdf_files/HASCAS%20Executive%20Summary2.pdf (accessed June 2010).

Taylor N (2008) Obstacles and dilemmas in the delivery of direct payments to service users with poor mental health. *Practice: Social Work in Action* **20** (1) 43–55.

Thornicroft G (2006) *Shunned: Discrimination against people with mental illness*. Oxford: Oxford University Press.

Time to Change (2008) *Stigma Shout: Service user and carer experiences of stigma and discrimination* [online]. Available at: http://www.rethink.org/how_we_can_help/campaigning_for_change/time_to_change/stigma_shout.html?shortcut=stigmashout (accessed June 2010).

Time to Change (2009) *Stigma of Mental Health Makes Finding Work in Recession More Difficult* [online]. Available at: http://www.time-to-change.org.uk/news/stigma-mental-health-makes-finding-work-recession-more-difficult-research-finds (accessed June 2010).

Verhaeghe M, Bracke P & Bruynooghe K (2007) Stigmatisation in different mental health services: a comparison of psychiatric and general hospitals. *Journal of Behavioural Health Services and Research* **34** (2) 186–197.

Wildman J (2003) Income related inequalities in mental health in Great Britain: analysing the causes of health inequality over time. *Journal of Health Economics* **22** (2) 295–312.

Section 5: Promoting recovery

Working in partnership to provide care and treatment that enables service users and carers to tackle mental health problems with hope and optimism and to work towards a valued lifestyle within and beyond the limits of any mental health problem.

Recovery approaches within mental health have received significant attention over the last decade, with recovery principles underpinning the future of services and support, as set out in the *New Horizons* consultation document.

> *'In a high-quality service, the principles of recovery and the concepts of hope, self-determination and opportunity that come under its umbrella underpin the practice of all those offering care and treatment.'* (DH, 2009, p24).

While it is not clear what the future direction of support services will be following the next general election and in the context of economic pressures, there are common themes that can be seen across service developments. Hope, choice and control are all aspects that are embedded in the future of mental health care, and having an understanding of how personalised services can promote these aspects can be helpful for both workers and service users while working towards recovery.

Aims

This section of the workbook will assist workers, service users and carers to consider how personalisation can promote and support recovery approaches. The overall aims of this section are:

- to link the areas of recovery and personalisation
- to develop understanding of recovery focused personalised support plans
- to consider wider social opportunities and the development of social capital to promote recovery.

Overview

The personalisation and recovery approaches are complementary. When planning, developing and delivering personalised services the individual's recovery should be central to the process, and aspects such as diversity and the multiple needs that individuals may have should be considered throughout this competence. For practitioners, developing competency in this area will assist them to understand and apply the two key agendas in mental health social care.

Eight areas of competence are included within this fifth shared capability, these are:

Competence 1:	Understand that recovery is a process that is unique to each person.
Competence 2:	Understand the essential role of hope in the recovery process.
Competence 3:	Accept that recovery is not about the elimination of symptoms or the notion of cure.
Competence 4:	Understand that the planning, arrangement and delivery of support should be determined by the needs of the service user.
Competence 5:	Work in a way that is flexible and responds to the expressed needs of the person.
Competence 6:	Ensure that all efforts are made to present non-stigmatising and positive views of people who experience mental health problems.
Competence 7:	Engage with external advocacy bodies to ensure that the rights and interests of service users are protected.
Competence 8:	Facilitate access to community groups and networks that enable the service user to participate in community activities.

By working through these competencies it will be possible to relate recovery approaches directly to the personalisation approach to inform practice. For service users and carers, working through this section will increase awareness of personalised care and consider how it can be used to promote individual recovery.

Competence 1

Understand that recovery is a process that is unique to each person.

Defining recovery has been an area of debate for many years, and it remains an area that is difficult to objectively measure. The personal nature of the recovery journey means that each individual's experience is unique and recovery is personally defined. One definition that has been influential within the area is that set out by Anthony in 1993 who stated that recovery was:

> *'...a deeply personal, unique process of changing one's attitudes, values, feelings, goals, skills and/or roles. It is a way of living a satisfying, hopeful, and contributing life even with limitations caused by the illness. Recovery involves the development of new meaning and purpose in one's life as one grows beyond the catastrophic effects of mental illness.'* (Anthony, 1993, p17)

This definition has been the basis of a wide range of studies and explorations of the recovery process, and it emphasises the range of experiences by placing recovery in the context of an individual's life rather than as an objective symptom based measurement.

Recovery can also be seen as going beyond social recovery to a full recovery, as set out by the Recovery In-sight team, who suggest that recovery is:

> *'...not only a social recovery and a growth through the breakdown, it also represents a growing mastering of illness management with resultant reduction of symptoms ie. full recovery.'* (www.recoveryin-sight.com)

The Recovery In-sight model includes training modules for individuals experiencing mental health problems, specifically bipolar disorder, that cover mood management techniques, healthy lifestyle choices, skills development, healthy lifestyle structure and balance, goal-planning and planning for sustained wellness. Evaluation of this approach shows positive outcomes for participants (Straughan & Buckenham, 2006).

Other definitions that have been set out within the policy arena and literature include:

> *'...a broad vision of recovery that involves a process of changing one's orientation and behaviour from a negative focus on a troubling event, condition or circumstance to the positive restoration, rebuilding, reclaiming or taking control of one's life.'*
> (NIMHE, 2005, p1)

> *'The experience of personal recovery can occur in the context of continuing symptoms or disabilities ... fundamentally (it) is about recovery of hope and ambition for living full and purposeful lives whatever the circumstances.'* (RCP/SCIE, 2007, p2)

The concept of the term recovery has been well debated, with questions raised as to whether the term itself is appropriate (SPN, 2007), with the different views and opinions of what constitutes recovery making it difficult to apply a consistent model to service delivery.

From a personalisation perspective, the individuality of recovery can be a useful framework as it encourages a holistic approach to the person's needs and wishes and enables a more creative view of what may be helpful to support and empower them to take control of their own situation, all areas which are central to the personalisation approach.

Question

What is your personal definition of recovery?

While there is a range of suggested definitions that demonstrate the diversity of the recovery experience, there are themes that emerge throughout which need to be considered when planning support that is recovery focused and personal to the individual.

Recovery themes

(developed from Shepherd *et al*, 2008; Davidson, 2008; NIMHE, 2005; Andresen *et al*, 2003)

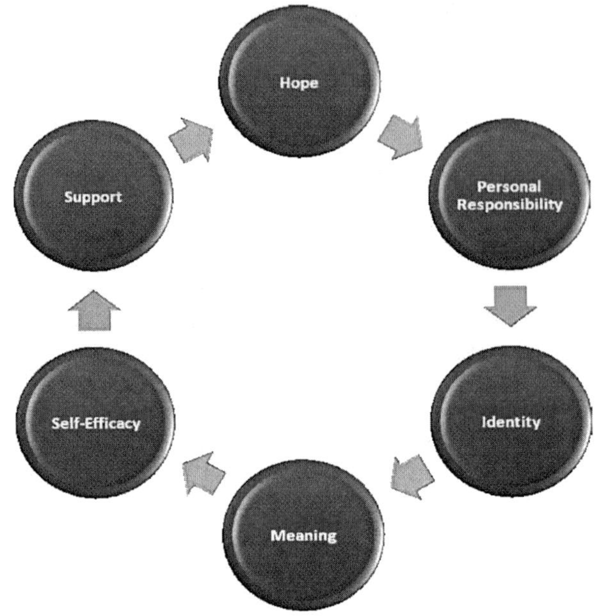

It is important to consider these areas within an individual's life in order to promote recovery. The individual and their context can be equally important in terms of positive outcomes and the person's recovery journey.

Case study

Sharon has been in and out of mental health services for the past five years; she has a care co-ordinator in the community and has had several admissions to the acute hospital. Her psychiatrist sees her on a bi-monthly basis and has prescribed a number of medications but Sharon feels the side effects of these are worse than the symptoms she experiences when she is unwell. Sharon has a diagnosis of bipolar disorder but does not agree with this diagnosis. She has previously received talking therapy in the form of cognitive behavioural approaches and has found self-help books to be helpful.

Before becoming unwell Sharon was a teacher at the local college, teaching marketing and sales at diploma level. She gave up her job when she was admitted to hospital for the first time as she felt unable to continue and said her employer was not supporting her. She has been claiming benefits since this time but says she feels like she has no purpose now and doesn't know what to do with her days.

Sharon is 34 years old, she is single and has two sisters, one of which lives nearby. She stays in contact with one of her friends from college but does not like to go out much as she feels people are judging her for being ill. Before her illness she enjoyed live music and learnt to play the piano, she also used to provide individual tuition for students in basic skills.

Questions to consider

- What aspects of Sharon's situation support the six key themes of recovery?
- What resources does Sharon have to draw upon to promote her own recovery?
- What are the potential barriers?

Competence 2

Understand the essential role of hope in the recovery process.

Hope is a central premise of recovery approaches. For an individual to start on the journey they need to believe that it is possible for them. It is more than just being well but rather a belief that the individual can lead a meaningful life. This belief develops over time and with encouragement, and may not be the key focus for individuals experiencing acute distress. The aim, whether as a practitioner, informal supporter or service user, is to create an environment in which hope can develop – for some this is a spiritual or religious experience, for others it is simply setting and reaching small goals that are achievable and then reflecting and learning from these. Approaches such as self-help, peer support and recovery stories are some of the means by which hope can be supported. Individuals need to believe that there are possibilities open to them in terms of their life chances and opportunities, and taking control of their own situations and learning from other's experiences are some ways in which this can be achieved. Research has demonstrated that individual hope is an essential factor if recovery is to be achieved (Ahern & Fisher, 2001; Mosher, 1999; Fisher & Chamberlin, 2004).

Personalisation and recovery both support social inclusion as a means to promote well-being. It is well established that aspects such as housing, employment, social contact, and leisure activities can all contribute to the promotion of the individual's quality of life and sense of control over their own situation (SEU, 2004; HM Government, 2009; Perkins *et al*, 2009; DH, 2009). The focus of traditional mental health services has been on clinical intervention and treatment, however, as mental illness is often unpredictable in terms of responses to treatment, it can be detrimental to supporting a sense of hope in the person. Considering and developing the wider context of the individual and their resources can help to focus on issues that are wider than symptoms and diagnosis, and can contribute to the sense of hope. This should include diversity issues beyond that of the mental health issue and encompass areas such as culture, ethnicity, faith, age and sexuality wherever this is relevant to the individual.

A number of studies have shown that self-management has a significant impact on the individual's recovery from mental health conditions (Allott *et al*, 2002; Rogers & Rogers, 2004; Copeland, 2004), and personalisation encourages this with choice and control for the individual as a fundamental component of the approach.

Reflection point

Considering your own situation, aims and aspirations, what gives you hope that you can achieve your goals?

Competence 3

Accept that recovery is not about the elimination of symptoms or the notion of cure.

The recovery approach has been developing throughout the history of mental health treatment and is not a new concept. Many of the principles of recovery received attention as a result of the user/survivor movement during the 1980s, which provided a challenge to professional power, and was underpinned by civil rights concepts such as self-help, empowerment and advocacy. In addition, a range of therapeutic communities, self-help addiction programmes, and support groups have all used the concept for many years, and these provide the foundations for what we know of recovery today (Shepherd *et al*, 2008).

Viewing recovery as being more than symptom-free or cured is a significant consideration. Mental health has traditionally been a medical model dominated field, however, over the last two decades, the social model has become more prominent and research evidence has been developed which shows that symptom control is only one element of the individual's situation that contributes to a sense of recovery and a better quality of life.

Best practice and research in the area of recovery may be based on variations, in terms of definition, however, the basic principles of all the evidence is that recovery is social and psychological as well as physiological, and continuation of symptoms does not necessarily result in poor outcomes for the individual. (Allott, 2002; Frese *et al*, 2001; Kelly & Gamble, 2005; Townsend & Glasser, 2003; Young & Ensing, 1999; Deegan, 1996; Anthony, 1993; Sullivan, 1997). From both the research evidence and individual user accounts, recovery in mental health appears to rest on the following principles.

- It is a holistic view of mental illness that focuses on the person, not just the symptoms and issues of human diversity need to be considered.
- It is achievable and can occur even though symptoms may reoccur.
- Individuals are responsible for the solution, not the problem.
- A well-organised support system is required to support recovery.
- Consumer rights, advocacy, and social change are all important aspects of recovery.

Reflection point

How do the principles of recovery support personalisation?

Competence 4

Understand that the planning, arrangement and delivery of support should be determined by the needs of the service user.

The initial *Putting People First* (DH, 2007b) document set out a requirement for a greater emphasis on self-assessment for social care needs, and is one of the elements of personalisation that will have a significant impact upon how services and support plans are organised and delivered. This emphasis wholly supports the recovery approach as it places the individual's lived experience as central to the assessment process. However, there remain barriers to this approach from frontline practitioners and service providers as risk remains a concern within the mental health arena. While there remains a need for professional assessment in mental health, and issues such as compulsory treatment and risk management need full consideration, this does not mean that the individual is unable to identify their own needs, and positive risk and risk sharing between user and worker need to be explored and developed to promote a greater emphasis on user control (Morgan, 2004; DH, 2007a; Langan & Lindow, 2004; Morgan, 2007).

The self-assessment process enables a higher level of involvement and control for the service user than has traditionally been available and places an emphasis on it within support planning and service delivery. This approach has been applied to mental health for a number of years, mainly in the form of wellness recovery action planning (WRAP), which has been shown to be very effective in terms of promoting and supporting individual recovery (Copeland, 1997).

WRAP is separated into five key areas that combined create an individual strengths assessment and a resource to support and maintain individual recovery, these are:

- wellness toolbox: identifying the strengths, supports and resources that the person has
- maintenance plan: setting out the routines and activities – daily, weekly and less frequently – that help the person to stay well
- early warning signs and identification of triggers: signs and symptoms that suggest the person is not as well as they could be and triggers that can cause difficulties and feelings of distress, including a plan for each of these areas to manage the impact
- crisis planning: setting out what the person would like to happen if they become unwell, the supports and measures they want to help them
- post-crisis planning: a plan to help a person recuperate after being unwell.

The WRAP process is a person-centred option that is available and well-evidenced within mental health recovery processes, and can be used within the personalisation context. Self-assessment and user involvement in support planning, which this competency supports, is central to WRAP and other forms of self-help. (Further information and training on WRAP is available from www.mentalhealthrecovery.com). It must be noted, however, that WRAP is not the only support planning tool, other approaches, such as the Recovery In-sight model, which focuses on developing a healthier lifestyle, building life skills (including coping techniques), and developing tools for improved living, can also provide a solid foundation for self-management and support planning (further information and training on the In-sight model is available from www.recoveryin-sight.com).

Personal budgets are a further way to support this competence. Once an individual has a need identified that requires social care support, the option for an individual or personal budget becomes available. The experience of the use of direct payments in mental health has been discouraging so far, with limited access from the mental health field (NIMHE, 2006), and this must be addressed if personalisation and user-led recovery is to be achieved within mental health care. The message from both central government and regional development centres is that mental health personal budgets and personalised support is an area that must be developed, and this is supported by SCIE, ADASS and the user/carer movements overall.

This requires professionals and practitioners to address the risk averse nature of current services and commissioners need to encourage far greater engagement from community groups, user-led organisations and mainstream universal services. This is a culture shift for traditional services and one that may be resisted. The role of users, carers and practitioners is to reject and challenge the view that mental health is 'too risky', and consider ways that personal budgets can be used to promote recovery for the individual.

The difference between direct payments, personal budgets and individual budgets is one area that has created difficulties within service delivery, and can contribute to the concerns about risk management. A recent parliamentary question discussed this issue, where Philip Hope, MP (Minister for Health) stated that:

> *'The terms individual budget and personal budget were used synonymously during the pilot stage of the personalisation project. However, personal budget is the term now being used for national implementation and relates to social care funding only. Individual budgets is now the term used for a notional amount of funding from a variety of sources which may include social care funding as well as other sources.'* (Hope, 2010)

To clarify this issue the definitions of each of these possible support packages are as follows.

- **Direct payments –** These are cash payments made to the individual assessed as needing a social care service (or their representative in cases where the person lacks capacity to manage the payments), in lieu of social care services. This cash amount must be used to purchase the required service directly.
- **Personal budgets –** This is the amount of money available to meet the assessed need. It is made up of the amount eligible for social care. The personal budget can either be paid to the individual (or their representative) or be managed by the provider or local authority, or be a combination of the two.
- **Individual budgets –** These are the total amount of funding available from across the range of funding streams – including social care, supporting people, disabled facilities grants, independent living funds, access to work and community equipment services.

In terms of personalisation in social care it will be direct payments or personal budgets that are currently available for users of mental health services to purchase and manage their support plans and services.

Case study exercise

Robert has been using mental health services for 10 years. He is under the care of a community mental health team and his care co-ordinator is a social worker employed by the local partnership trust. His care programme approach assessment and care plan identified a number of social needs that he would need support with, and a plan has been put together to meet these needs. He is not currently receiving a direct payment or personal budget. His agreed needs include the following.

- **Social contact –** Robert is quite isolated and when unwell tends to withdraw from contact even further. His care co-ordinator has arranged weekly contact with a support worker to take him out, and two courses at the day centre each week – cooking class and football club. He would also like to access his local faith group.
- **Vocation –** Robert was referred to the employment support project run by the mental health trust but he found this unhelpful. He is a qualified electrician, but has not worked for 12 years and is finding it difficult to re-enter employment.

- **Activity –** A membership at the local leisure centre has been arranged, but this is several miles from Robert's home and public transport is only available twice a day (early morning and tea time).

Task

Identify the possible personalisation options – including the use of direct payments or personal budgets, to support Robert.

Competence 5

Work in a way that is flexible and responds to the expressed needs of the person.

Both structural and cultural/practice issues need to be considered within this competency. One of the key developments that the National Service Framework (DH, 1999) supported, and which *New Horizons* (DH, 2009) and personalisation will continue, was the 24/7 access to services, and more activity-based services available at times that suit the individual.

As with other public services, mental health care has traditionally expected service users to fit in with the set structure with organisations dictating how, where and when, services are delivered. However, the emphasis on recovery, which includes a range of social and community-based involvement, and the development and delivery of person-centred care means that these traditional structures have no option other than to change and respond to the demands of those who use the services.

Personal budgets provide the facility for individuals to purchase their own support, and with this comes the ability to state what and when is needed. Services will increasingly need to adapt to this shift if they are to survive in the marketplace. As with any consumer market – if the service cannot meet the demands of the person buying it the person will go elsewhere. In addition, tools such as self-assessment, advanced statements and directives and WRAP plans all respond flexibly to the needs of a person coming into mental health services. There is a need for both users and workers to have an awareness of the range of options available to them. There are a number of examples of how direct payments and personal budgets can be used creatively to promote and support recovery, for example, research by Spandler & Vick (2006) highlighted possibilities such as employing a personal assistant to accompany individuals to access leisure, community and household support.

One particular issue to consider and challenge is the concept of risk, which in mental health services can be a significant barrier to user choice and control. Positive risk is something that has been talked about in mental health terms for some time (Morgan, 2004; DH, 2007a; Slade, 2009), however, it seems that the potential of this approach has not been realised. There remains a tendency for workers to remain risk averse and protective rather than promote the user's right to take risks. This is one of the factors that was identified in terms of the reasons for lower take-up in mental health of direct payments (PSSRU, 2007; Newbigging & Lowe, 2003; Leadbetter *et al*, 2008; Coldham *et al*, 2005), and remains a cultural issue to overcome in mental health services.

Exercise

- What are the benefits and potential risks of providing a personal budget and direct payment for a person in the following situation and how can these be minimised?

As part of his agreed support plan, Robert joins an art class. He needs approximately £120 to pay for materials and would benefit from a personal assistant to support him – he applies for a one-off direct payment for his costs and uses a personal budget to employ a personal assistant.

Multiple needs and identities must to be noted at this point – it is often the case that an individual has a range of identities and roles that they fulfil in their lives. These relate to both how the person perceives themself and how they relate to others in their social circumstances and relationship. A personalised support plan needs to consider the full range of roles and identities if it is to be truly person-centred and meaningful to the individual. Social roles can include family roles – son, daughter, parent, spouse, sibling, grandparent – as well as friend, employee, student or other relationship. Identities usually relate to how the individual sees themselves and will have a social or cultural meaning, for example, identification with a particular ethnicity, faith, sexuality or age group. Assessment and support planning will need to explore these areas and identify any information, advice or support that would benefit the individual or which they would like to access as part of their goal setting and support planning process.

Example

Ajay is a 24-year-old Muslim man. He lives at home with his parents and two sisters who are both younger than him. His parents immigrated to the UK in the 1970s and are originally from Pakistan. Ajay's parents are now saying that it is time he considers getting married and have introduced him to several women from the community. He has recently told his friend that he is gay, but is struggling with how this will be received by his family and is experiencing a high degree of guilt as his religion does not accept homosexuality and his parents are expecting him to get married and have children.

- A number of roles and identities are present in Ajay's case – he is a Muslim, a member of the Pakistani community, a son, a gay man, a brother and a friend. His identities are not complementary and his needs will include helping him to come to terms with his sexuality and supporting him to make decisions around whether he is to talk to his parents about his sexuality and the possible consequences of this. Specific black and minority ethnic (BME) advocacy may be needed and local lesbian, gay, bisexual and transgender (LGBT) support would help him to work through some of his concerns.

Competence 6

Ensure that all efforts are made to present non-stigmatising and positive views of people who experience mental health problems.

Reducing the stigma that surrounds mental health difficulties is a barrier that individuals face on a daily basis in terms of the recovery and personalisation journey. Social inclusion and community involvement are both areas that have been shown to increase the person's likelihood of recovery from severe mental health problems (Rogers & Rogers, 2004; SEU, 2004) and key to implementing personalisation within mental health. The role of universal services is highlighted as one of the key areas that needs to be developed to increase choice and improve equality of access, and there is a need to think beyond what is provided by traditional mental health services for competency to be developed in this area.

What are universal services?

This means that everyone, no matter what their age, ability, disability or difference, can access their local public and commercial services such as transport, information, advice and advocacy, housing, primary health care (GPs etc), leisure centres, schools and libraries. The universal services part of personalisation aims to make sure that everyone can access the same services.

Addressing and challenging stigma is an area that has been widely considered and debated, and while there has been significant progress, there remains a public and media based view of mental illness as something that is to be feared. This is unhelpful as it serves to continue the exclusion of people within our society, and is detrimental to personal well-being. Challenging the prejudices and stereotypes associated with mental health is a huge task, and many projects and campaigns have (and continue) to contribute to breaking down some of the barriers. The competency for workers in this area is to challenge views as they encounter them, and to facilitate access to universal services for general health and social needs wherever possible. Focusing on the element of hope, which is central to both recovery and personalisation, requires service users and carers to believe that it is possible to achieve their goals, and negative views can have a significant impact. An individual has far more to offer than just their mental health status, and this needs to be considered and promoted both within mental health care and in the wider social context.

Reflection point

What are some of the labels and roles that apply to you? How do they impact on how others treat and respond to you?

Competence 7

Engage with external advocacy bodies to ensure that the rights and interests of service users are protected.

Advocacy can be defined as the process of one person or group speaking out on behalf of another person or group, with the aim being to influence the outcomes that directly affect that person or group (Cohen *et al*, 2001). Advocacy services are available in all local areas, and it is one of the facilities available for people to ensure they are treated fairly, with proper consideration of needs, wishes, options and rights.

Advocacy and support services for specific groups are also available in most areas, for example BME and LGBT advocacy services, which are often run by members of the communities they serve and who have a thorough understanding of the multiple issues that may face members of these groups.

There is a range of advocacy services and roles – some general and some with specific legal duties. Ensuring that people have the right information about these is an important competency for practitioners across health and social care.

Advocacy roles

- **Independent mental capacity advocate (IMCA)**
  A statutory role under the Mental Capacity Act (2005), the IMCA role is to ensure that the rights of a person who lacks capacity to make a specific decision are safeguarded.
- **Independent mental health advocate (IMHA)**
  A statutory role under the Mental Health Act (2007), the IMHA role is to represent the rights of an individual who has been detained under the Mental Health Act and ensure that the safeguards and the principles of the act are provided to the person.
- **Independent complaints advocacy service (ICAS)**
  An advocacy service specifically created to support individuals who are making complaints about NHS care or services. The ICAS role is to support the person and ensure that the NHS procedures are carried out properly.
- **Mental health and general advocacy**
  There is a range of advocacy services, both user-led and commissioned from voluntary sector organisations, in mental health and also more general. The role for these advocates is supporting the person concerned and ensuring that the individual's voice and views are represented and heard.
- **Specific groups advocacy**
  Advocacy services for (and often run by) members of specific groups. These can be both local and national organisations and are often user-led provisions. The main aim of these services is to provide support that takes into account the specific needs and cultural understandings of different groups.

Activity

Find out what services are provided in your area, collect the contact addresses and any available leaflets or information. What does each service provide?

Competence 8

Facilitate access to community groups and networks that enable the service user to participate in community activities.

Social capital and social inclusion are important parts of the personalisation agenda, as well as being key components of the recovery approach, and a central part of the policy direction for the future of mental health services (DH, 2009). As such, there needs to be an increased awareness, by those within the field, of the various groups, networks and resources that are available in each community area. Diversity and differing cultural needs also need to be acknowledged and groups such as faith groups, BME communities, and other group specific services that are operating in each locality need to be highlighted to both service users and providers.

Within the personalisation and recovery agenda an individual's support plan should be wider than just those services provided by mental health specific providers, and include universal services, community organisations and groups. This can include such diverse areas as learning and education, hobbies, sports and leisure, transport and travel, community volunteering, spiritual groups, and social clubs, as well as any other activities that are identified as a need or aspiration for the individual.

In this context, information itself becomes a service and the competency for the worker becomes being able to identify and facilitate access to the relevant group or network and support the individual to take part in these. The skills developed elsewhere in this competency – for example being able to challenge stigma and foster hope – are essential in the delivery of this area, as is a detailed awareness of the local area and facilities. A resource directory listing groups, networks, and organisations, including what each of these do or provide, can be a useful tool for both workers and users, however, these are only useful if they are current.

The worker needs to be able to think wider than what has traditionally been available and be creative in the support planning processes to include non-traditional groups, services and providers, this includes knowing where to find information (for example libraries, local papers etc), and be able to incorporate this local knowledge into their routine practice.

Exercise

Imagine you are working with the following users. What groups or resources in your local area could be accessed and what support may be needed to facilitate access?

Sarah has been watching 'Strictly Come Dancing' and wants to learn how to dance the waltz. She is a complete beginner. She is nervous around new people and has no one she can take with her. She experiences panic attacks.

Clive reads a lot, particularly crime and thrillers. He wants to talk to others about the books he reads and would like to join a book club. He has depression and finds it difficult to read books about mental health problems.

Salma is very active in the local Polish community. She has previously experienced periods of alcohol use and self-harm and would like to help others who are experiencing similar problems within her community.

Rachel feels she needs to lose weight but is struggling to stay motivated. She would like to join a class but struggles with men and large groups.

Darren wants to tell his family that he is gay, but is finding it difficult to talk to them because he is worried about how they will react. He has experienced depression and harmed himself on several occasions. He feels that he wants to meet people in the same situation but in a social setting that does not involve drinking alcohol.

Summary

This section has considered the competency of 'promoting recovery' within mental health and how that applies to the personalisation approach. The definition of this competency within the 10 Essential Shared Capabilities is:

> *'Working in partnership to provide care and treatment that enables service users and carers to tackle mental health problems with hope and optimism and to work towards a valued lifestyle within and beyond the limits of any mental health problem.'*

The competencies presented have demonstrated that personalisation, recovery and the wider social inclusion and involvement issues are complementary and workers need to develop an awareness of how these link and promote each other. The whole person approach requires workers to consider a range of social issues and to develop an in-depth knowledge of the resources and facilities, including the issues which are not traditionally mental health focused, in order to meet the needs and aspirations of the individual. Personalised support is a user-focused approach and developing competence in this area is key to delivering services that are transformational for those who experience mental health difficulties.

Summary exercise

Write a short summary of what this capability means to you in your context/practice, and then answer the following three questions.

- What have you learnt by completing this section?

- How have you now reached competence in this area?

- What do you need to do to maintain your competence?

References

Ahern L & Fisher DB (2001) Recovery at your own PACE (Personal Assistance in Community Existence). *Journal of Psychosocial Nursing* **24** 22–32.

Allott P (2002) Discovering hope for recovery from a British perspective: a review of a selection of recovery literature, implications for practice and systems change. In: S Lime, M McCubbin & B Dallgire (Eds) International Innovations in Community Mental Health (Special Issue). *Canadian Journal of Community Mental Health* **21** (3).

Allott P, Loganathan L & Fulford KWM (2002) Discovering hope for recovery. *Canadian Journal of Community Mental Health* **21** (2) 13–34.

Andresen R, Oades L & Caputi P (2003) The experience of recovery from schizophrenia: towards an empirically validated stage model. *Australian and New Zealand Journal of Psychiatry* **37** 586–594.

Anthony WA (1993) Recovery from mental illness: the guiding vision of the mental health service system in the 1990s. *Psychosocial Rehabilitation Journal* **16** (4) 11–23.

Cohen D, De la Vega R, & Watson G (2001) *Advocacy for Social Justice*. Bloomfield, CT: Kumarian Press Inc.

Coldham T, Newbigging K & Vick N (2005) Cash in their hands. *Mental Health Today* June, 26–29.

Copeland ME (1997) *WRAP–Wellness Recovery Action Plan*. Brattleboro, VT: Peach Press.

Copeland ME (2004) Self-determination in mental health recovery: taking back our lives. In: J Jonikas & J Cook (Eds) *UIC NRTC's National Self-Determination and Psychiatric Disability Invitational Conference: Conference Papers* (pp 68–82). Chicago, IL: UIC National Research and Training Center on Psychiatric Disability.

Davidson L (2008) *Recovery – Concepts and Application*. Devon Recovery Group. Available at: www.scmh.org.uk

Deegan P (1996) Recovery as a journey of the heart. *Psychiatric Rehabilitation Journal* **19** (3) 91–97.

Department of Health (1999) *National Service Framework for Mental Health*. London: TSO.

Department of Health (2007a) *Best Practice in Managing Risk: Principles and guidance for best practice in the assessment and management of risk to self and others in mental health services*. London: TSO.

Department of Health (2007b) *Putting People First: A shared vision and commitment to adult social care*. London: TSO.

Department of Health (2009) *New Horizons: Towards a shared vision for mental health – consultation*. London: TSO.

Fisher D & Chamberlin J (2004) *Personal Assistance in Community Existence: Recovery through peer support*. Lawrence, Mass: National Empowerment Center.

Frese FJ, Stanley J, Kress K & Vogel-Scibilia S (2001) Integrating evidence-based practices and the recovery model. *Psychiatric Services* **52** 11 1462–1468.

Hope P (2010) Hansard - HC Deb, 18 January 2010, c115W.

HM Government (2009) *Work, Recovery and Inclusion*. London: TSO.

Kelly M & Gamble C (2005) Exploring the concept of recovery in schizophrenia. *Journal of Psychiatric and Mental Health Nursing* **12** (2) 245–251.

Langan J & Lindow V (2004) *Living with Risk: Mental health service user involvement in risk assessment and management*. Bristol: Polity Press/Joseph Rowntree Foundation.

Leadbetter C, Bartlett J & Gallagher N (2008) *Making it Personal*. London: Demos.

Morgan S (2004) Positive risk-taking: an idea whose time has come. *Health Care Risk Report* October 18–19.

Morgan S (2007) Working with risk. *Mental Health Today* Sept 36–37.

Mosher L (1999) Soteria House and other alternatives to acute psychiatric hospitalization. *Journal of Nervous and Mental Disease* **187** 142–147.

Newbigging K & Lowe J (2003) *Implementing Direct Payments in Mental Health*. York: Joseph Rowntree Foundation.

NIMHE (2005) *Guiding Statement on Recovery*. London: DH.

NIMHE (2006) *Direct Payments for People with Mental Health Problems: A guide to action*. London: TSO.

Perkins R, Farmer P & Litchfield P (2009) *Realising Ambition: Better employment support for people with a mental health condition*. London: TSO.

PSSRU (2007) *Direct Payments: A national survey of direct payments policy and practice*. London: LSE PSSRU.

RCP/SCIE (2007) *A Common Purpose: Recovery in future mental health services*. London: SCIE.

Rogers J & Rogers S (2004) Self-determination for people with psychiatric disabilities: Personal obstacles and facilitators. In: J Jonikas & JA Cook (Eds) *UIC NRTC's National Self-Determination and Psychiatric Disability Invitational Conference: Conference Papers* (pp 7–23). Chicago, IL: UIC National Research and Training Center on Psychiatric Disability.

Shepherd G, Boardman J & Slade M (2008) *Making Recovery a Reality*. London: Sainsbury Centre for Mental Health.

Slade M (2009) *100 Ways to Support Recovery: A guide for mental health professionals*. Rethink recovery series volume 1. London: Rethink. Available at: http://www.rethink.org/100ways

Social Exclusion Unit (2004) *Mental Health and Social Exclusion*. TSO: London.

Spandler H & Vick N (2006) Opportunities for independent living using direct payments in mental health. *Health and Social Care in the Community* **14** (2) 107–115.

SPN (2007) *Whose Recovery Is It Anyway?* Paper 11. London: SPN. Available at: http://www.spn.org.uk/fileadmin/SPN_uploads/Documents/Papers/SPN_Papers/Recovery_and_Diversity_Booklet.pdf

Sullivan WP (1997) A long and winding road: the process of recovery from severe mental illness. In: L Spaniol, C Gagne & M Koehler (Eds) *Psychological and Social Aspects of Psychiatric Disability*. Boston: Center for Psychiatric Rehabilitation.

Straughan H & Buckenham M (2006) In-sight: an evaluation of user-led, recovery-based, holistic group training for bipolar disorder. *Journal of Public Mental Health* **5** (3) 29–43.

Townsend W & Glasser N (2003) Recovery: The heart and soul of treatment. *Psychiatric Rehabilitation Journal* **27** (1) 83–86.

Young SL & Ensing DS (1999) Exploring recovery from the perspective of people with psychiatric disabilities. *Psychiatric Rehabilitation Journal* **22** (3) 219–231.

Section 6: Identifying people's needs and strengths

Working in partnership to gather information to agree health and social care needs in the context of the preferred lifestyle and aspirations of service users, their families, carers and friends.

As already emphasised throughout this workbook, the individual is central to all support processes, and personalisation provides a framework and mechanism through which this can be achieved. This section concentrates on identifying an individual's needs and strengths. The strengths approach is a way of working with people, which is rooted in the social model of disability, and is based upon highlighting people's ability to make changes and take control of their own situations (McCashen, 2005).

One study that highlighted a strengths-based approach to recovery and mental health well-being was carried out across 10 European countries during 2007–2008 by Turton *et al* (2010). This study surveyed stakeholder groups of service users, professionals, carers and advocates, to attempt to identify the things they felt were important to recovery. A range of areas was identified, including social inclusion, self-management, staff attitudes and level of autonomy. The importance of a whole-person, strengths-based approach to treatment was also emphasised, alongside choices concerning meaningful occupation and a range of talking therapies.

Aims

This section of the workbook will assist workers, service users and carers to identify the strengths as well as the needs of the person and incorporate these into their day-to-day practice. The overall aims of the section are:

- to create a direct link between an individual's strengths and resources and how these can influence recovery
- to link personalisation and personal strengths to promote choice and control within support systems
- to provide an awareness of how the social model of mental health can be applied to understand and engage with wider social systems.

Overview

Every individual who accesses mental health services brings with them unique needs and a range of strengths and resources on which they can draw. This competence is designed to assist readers to identify these and plan support based on an awareness of the full range of social factors that can have an impact on an individual's well-being. This is not a process that is done in isolation: the individual's context, wishes and preferences and their support network can all be drawn upon to develop partnerships between services, the person and their community, and as such, the principles of a personalised approach, based on individual needs and strengths is consistent with strengths-based approaches.

Five areas of competence are included within this first shared capability, these are:

Competence 1:	Carry out (or contribute to) a systematic, whole systems assessment that has as its focus the strengths and needs of the service user and those family and friends who support them.
Competence 2:	Work in a way that acknowledges the personal, social, cultural and spiritual strengths and needs of the individual.
Competence 3:	Understand how the physical and mental health of an individual can be promoted or demoted and the impact that an individual's health needs, mental or physical, may have on other parts of the system.
Competence 4:	Understand the impact that other parts of the system may have on the individual's physical and mental health.
Competence 5:	Work in partnership with the individual's support network to collect information to assist understanding of the person and their strengths and needs.

From a personalisation perspective these competencies form the basis of co-production as they draw upon the resources of both the individual and the various support mechanisms to build a support package delivered in partnership. These partnerships also enable choice and control by the person as their lifestyle preferences and aspirations are the goals that drive the support.

By working through these competencies the reader will be able to identify and incorporate an individual's needs and strengths into the personalisation approach, and understand how these strengths and resources support an individual's recovery.

Competence 1

Carry out (or contribute to) a systematic, whole systems assessment that has as its focus the strengths and needs of the service user and those family and friends who support them.

Within adult services, including mental health, focusing on the service user is central to the assessment and support processes. It can be counterproductive to work with an individual without considering their social support network and systems, as needs may be missed. No individual exists within a vacuum; they interact with a range of people, groups, and services as part of daily life, and these interactions can be both positive and negative in terms of the individual's well-being.

Systems: the range of possible social involvements and interactions

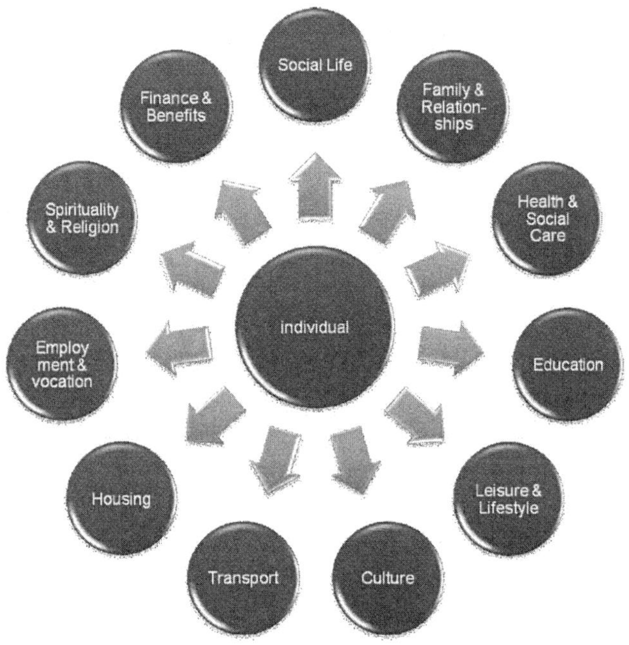

The aim of the diagram above is to provide an overview of some of the areas that may make up a person's interactions and contacts. It is not exhaustive and people will have more or less involvement with the range of areas highlighted depending upon their individual situation and lifestyle. However, each individual will have a system in which they operate and their needs and strengths may have a much wider impact than just upon the individual in isolation.

Personalisation highlights social capital as a key element of the approach, and this means that support plans need to consider carers, families and wider social contacts alongside the person. Carer assessments may be a more common element with mental health services, however, many individuals who support individuals with mental health difficulties do not view themselves as carers (NMHDU, 2010), or may not be suitable for an assessment as the caring role is more distant than the immediate supports available to the person. To be able to develop and draw upon social capital within the individual's circumstances, the assessment and planning processes need to consider the person's whole system and the resources they have to draw upon, including those beyond traditional services and linking into communities and local groups (Glendinning *et al*, 2005).

Case study exercise

Gary is 23 years old. He was a student at the local university studying geography until about six months ago when he started to experience strange things happening to him. He describes it as not being able to tell what was real. He became anxious and depressed as a result of these experiences and eventually withdrew from his course. He has deferred his final year but says he does want to finish it at some point in the future. He has a good relationship with his personal tutor who has supported his deferment and he has also been seeing a support worker provided by the university's student support service. He can only have another month of contact now that he has officially deferred his course.

Gary has been living in a shared house with three other students. He went to stay with his parents a few weeks ago but wants to return to the shared house. His brother, Dermot, is a year older than him and is working in the city where Gary was at university. The two are close and regularly go out around town and to bars and clubs together. Gary's housemates want him to return to the house but are concerned that they will not be able to support him and would like some information and support around what they should and should not be doing. Gary's parents, however, think he should stay at home as they can look after him better.

Gary has been involved with a few groups with the university student union, including the men's hockey club, and he wants to keep up with hockey once he is feeling better. Gary is also a member of the local church, however, he has not been there since he started having his strange experiences as he is worried what people will think.

Questions

- Identify Gary's support network.
- What are the strengths and needs of Gary and his support network highlighted in the information presented?
- What would be the initial support plan for Gary?

Competence 2

Work in a way that acknowledges the personal, social, cultural and spiritual strengths and needs of the individual.

Every person is unique, with an individual set of beliefs, needs, cultures and strengths. These are based on experiences, perceptions and values, all of which develop both in response to social situations and interactions and as a result of a person's psychological understanding of their environment (Anthony, 1993; Taylor & Brown, 1988; Owen & Khalil, 2007). Within this context it is necessary to consider personal, social, cultural and spiritual elements as part of the assessment and support planning processes to make sure that services are appropriate to the person and their situation, meets their diverse needs, and builds on the strengths they possess.

Within the guidance around addressing and responding to diversity, six strands are identified, these are – age, gender, sexuality, disability, race and religion or belief. Support services need to ensure that their activities are inclusive and appropriate and that they are able to acknowledge an individual's strengths and needs in these areas. There are some key risk factors associated with certain groups, for example, LGBT people have a much higher risk of developing mental health difficulties, along with a higher rate of suicide, self-harm and substance misuse than the general population (DH, 2007; NIMHE, 2007). Additionally, it has been shown that staff and service responses to LGBT needs are insensitive and can be hostile (Fish, 2009; Fish, 2007; DH, 2007; PACE, 2008). In some extreme cases professionals have even tried to change them into heterosexuals (Bartlett *et al*, 2009; MacFarlane, 1998).

Examples of negative attitudes, or services which do not respond to particular needs, could be found across the diversity strands, and it seems that services and workers need to pay closer attention to personal, social, cultural and spiritual needs and strengths, if they are to support the individual's recovery in a personalised way.

Personalisation provides a real opportunity for services and workers to develop ways in which the needs and strengths of diverse people can be addressed and promoted. Whether needs and strengths are associated with sexuality, gender, race or other factors, personal budgets and direct payments can be used to purchase support that enables the person to take part in a lifestyle that they choose, and help community organisations and groups to provide support that is not available from the more traditional services (CSCI, 2008; Cocker & Hafford-Letchfield, 2010; Allen *et al*, 2009; Manthorpe & Bowes, 2010).

Case study

Caroline is a 25-year-old woman from an Evangelical church family. She has been active in church life since she was a small child and has many friends through this group. Caroline went to college when she left school and qualified as a beautician. She has worked on and off over the last few years and she is currently working two days a week at a local salon.

Caroline has been in contact with mental health services for the past few years as she has periods of depression and anxiety and can become very obsessive. She sees her psychiatrist regularly. About a year ago she told two of her close friends that she was gay. One of her friends was uncomfortable with this and said that while she didn't blame her for the feelings she could not accept a same-sex relationship as they felt it was sinful. Caroline took this reaction very hard and became very withdrawn.

Recently Caroline met a woman at work who she is attracted to and has been out for a meal with her on two occasions. Caroline wants to start a relationship with this woman but is struggling to come to terms with her friend's reaction and is scared that her family and other friends at the church will reject her as a result. Her other friend is being very supportive and is encouraging Caroline to see the woman again.

On attending an appointment with her psychiatrist recently, Caroline became very distressed. The psychiatrist has made a referral to the local mental health team as he feels she needs some additional support at the moment.

Questions

Imagine you are the case worker who has received the referral and is assessing Caroline's situation.

- What are the personal, social and spiritual needs in Caroline's case?
- What are Caroline's strengths and resources?
- How could a personalised approach support Caroline's strengths and needs?

Considering the spiritual aspects of mental health support has been identified as an area of good practice (Anthony, 1993; Mental Health Foundation, 2006; Sims & Cook, 2009). Historically, religion and spirituality have been part of understanding mental health issues, and there is no simple or fixed distinction between them, as the many episodes of 'voice hearing' in religious texts shows. However, this overlap in interpretation has not always been helpful, notably where a practitioner's own beliefs have been imposed on the individual. There are some extreme examples in the history of mental health care, such as people with psychosis and other issues being put through exorcism rituals (Sims & Cook, 2009; Boehnlein, 2000; Koenig, 2005).

From a personalisation perspective, the spiritual dimension of the person, including the consideration of their beliefs and practices, should be embedded within the assessment and support planning processes. Spirituality can contribute to a person's well-being, and also their individual identity. In order to have a truly personalised approach, spirituality is one of the elements that should be crucial to the person's support.

Competence 3

Understand how the physical and mental health of an individual can be promoted or demoted and the impact that an individual's health needs, mental or physical, may have on other parts of the system.

Mental health difficulties are not static; they fluctuate and change, and can be affected by a wide range of both internal and external forces. There are many studies that have been carried out into how social and psychological factors influence individual well-being and recovery (Young & Ensing, 1999; Shepherd *et al*, 2008; Allott *et al*, 2002). These include factors such as the support of family and friends, access to general health services, occupation, social interaction, as well as aspects such as how the individual copes and deals with stress, and their level of self-esteem.

At times when a person is struggling or unwell, the impact on their well-being and needs can have far reaching implications. An individual will interact with a wide range of people, and each person takes on a range of roles and identities. For example, someone can be a brother, a son, a husband, a friend and a worker. If the individual also has multiple identities, for example, is a member of a particular community or group due to ethnicity, sexuality, faith or other factors, these interactions and the influence one has on the other can become very complex and interdependent. In each relationship or connection that an individual has, they play a role, and the removal or disruption of that role can have a significant impact upon the social system.

The immediate family and any explicit caring relationships are often considered by support services, with carer assessment and support being a common feature of community services. *The Carers Strategy* published in 2008 (DH, 2008a) states that by 2018 all carers will be regarded as 'expert care partners' with access to integrated and personalised services to support their role.

> *'...by 2018, carers will be universally recognised and valued as being fundamental to strong families and stable communities. Support will be tailored to meet individuals' needs, enabling carers to maintain a balance between their caring responsibilities and a life outside caring, while enabling the person they support to be a full and equal citizen.'* (DH, 2008a, p16)

As a result, the immediate family of an individual who is experiencing mental distress is becoming increasingly involved in support planning. Local authorities include support and assessment for carers as a key performance target and it often forms a local area agreement (LAA) target for service improvement across public services in each area.

Local area agreements

Local area agreements (LAAs) are three-year action plans for achieving better outcomes, developed by councils with their partners in local strategic partnerships (LSP), such as PCTs, NHS trusts and third sector providers. LAAs for 2008–11 have been agreed with central government for all 150 local authority areas in England.

Each one has been negotiated with the relevant regional government office (GO), and includes a mix of national and local priorities and targets, relevant to the area. LAAs are the main way for central government and local services to work together. They also underpin the national performance framework and its priorities, through which central government measures progress.

The definition of a carer is a complex one, and people who provide informal support often do not see themselves as carers (NMHDU, 2010). The definition of a carer for the purposes of the carer's strategy is:

> *'A carer spends a significant proportion of their life providing unpaid support to family or potentially friends. This could be caring for a relative, partner or friend who is ill, frail, disabled or has mental health or substance misuse problems.'* (DH, 2008a, p19)

The wider social network is often disregarded by service providers, and while it is a positive step that carers and immediate family members are included and engaged, the extended family or community also needs to be considered if social capital is to become a reality in a personalised social care system.

Case study exercise

Alex is diagnosed with schizophrenia. He has been in contact with mental health services for 10 years and has had numerous inpatient admissions due to psychotic symptoms, which include hallucinations, delusions and paranoia. Alex hears several voices and these are usually telling him to hurt himself.

Alex is 31 and lives with his mother and stepfather. He has moved out on two previous occasions but struggled to keep his tenancies on both occasions and became very distressed as a result.

Alex has a brother and a sister. His sister lives locally with her husband and two children, she visits regularly and helps Alex with things like his benefits paperwork. Alex's brother is away at university, but Alex usually visits him once each term for a weekend. Alex spends a lot of time with a school friend who owns a local garage and gives him jobs to do, and his uncle who is retired and goes out with Alex twice a week.

Questions

- Who in this case study would be included in the definition of a carer?
- Who should be considered and engaged in the assessment process?
- What is the possible impact of changes to the supports that Alex receives?

Competence 4

Understand the impact that other parts of the system may have on the individual's physical and mental health.

As set out in section 5, there is a wide range of influences on an individual's well-being and mental health recovery journey, and these include the wider social and system factors. The social model of mental health sets out a clear understanding of the impact of social factors on the individual. This needs to be considered within this competence in order to develop an understanding of the approach and be able to respond appropriately to these needs.

According to research in the area, the social model in mental health has a number of key characteristics, these include the following.

- An understanding of the complexity of human health and well-being that emphasises the interaction of social factors with those of physical health and biology and considers the impact of these on health and disease.

- It addresses the inner and the outer worlds of individuals, groups and communities, and takes on the experiences and supports of the social networks of people. By working collaboratively within social institutions it seeks to promote the interests of individuals and communities and challenges where the system has negative effects.
- It emphasises shared knowledge and shared territory with a range of disciplines and with service users and the general public, and emphasises empowerment and capacity building at individual and community level by placing equal value on the expertise of service users, carers and the general public.
(Duggan *et al*, 2002, p19)

The social model is one way of understanding the impact that the social system can have on both an individual's overall mental health and their recovery (Beresford, 2002; Duggan *et al*, 2002). From a personalisation perspective the social system can have a significant impact on an individual's experience and the engagement of community and informal supports, as well as in areas such as employment and education.

Social isolation and lack of social support systems have been identified as key influences in mental health prevention and recovery (SEU, 2003; RCP/SCIE, 2007; DH, 2009), with better outcomes for people who have support networks that are engaged and involved in the support planning processes (SEU, 2003; Slade, 2009; Davidson, 2008). As such, workers need to be aware of these influences and the impact they may be having on the person.

Reflection exercise

Consider your own social network – people you see or have contact with daily, weekly and more occasionally.

- What impact would it have on your physical and mental well-being if you were not able to maintain this contact?

Consider the services and community activities/groups that you regularly access – including GPs or other primary care, education, employment, leisure activities, religious or BME communities and groups etc.

- What impact would it have on your physical and mental well-being if you were not able to access these services, groups or activities?

For the spirit of *Putting People First* (DH, 2008b) and subsequent guidance to be implemented there is a need for engagement across the whole range of systems. First, there needs to be an extension of information, advice and support across informal support networks, for example, supporting carers and communities, and developing social capital by strengthening the resources and building capacity within communities to provide support to individuals and families. Second, there needs to be organisational and professional arrangements, such as supporting universal services to provide appropriate support in the community setting, for example, primary care extending its services to include psychological therapies with specialist services supporting these developments.

Competence 5

Work in partnership with the individual's support network to collect information to assist understanding of the person and their strengths and needs.

While considering the person's social system and support network is necessary for a personalised approach and assessment process, working in partnership is also a key requirement. A large part of personalisation relies on partnerships, and engaging with support networks is one of the means by which a clearer picture of the person's circumstances and environment can be developed.

The needs and strengths of both the individual and their supports are linked together and often depend upon each other, and one should not be considered in isolation from the other if a truly personalised support plan is to be implemented.

Carer assessment and family work are just two of the means by which a person's support network can be accessed, however, there needs to be a sense of partnership rather than just a consultation for engagement to be meaningful for all concerned. The recent publication by the National Mental Health Development Unit (NMHDU, 2010) suggests some examples of how this can be achieved, which includes assessment systems and processes based on personalisation principles, and members of the support network being treated as equal partners to develop support. These elements are crucial to the personalisation approach, and services also need to listen and draw upon the information that the person's support network can provide.

A person's support network can be identified by looking at their average weekly activities and the people that they may come into contact with. The exercises in section 1 can assist with this task and help the person to set out what support they have and the roles of these. It is often the case that wider support is more difficult to identify and communities, groups, spirituality, leisure activities, employment and education are all possible areas where a person may access informal and ad hoc support. These areas supplement the immediate family, friends and any carer relationships that the person may have.

It must be remembered that services often only see an individual for a few hours a week, whereas family and friends are with the person for much longer periods of time, and may be able to provide intelligence in terms of what would be helpful and what could promote the person's recovery. This should always be done with the individual's agreement, and partnerships between services, the individual and their support system need to ensure that any issues in relation to confidentiality are addressed from the initial stages.

Case study exercise

Jack is 37 and married to Claire. He has experienced depression, anxiety, obsessional behaviour and periods where he has self-harmed for several years, and is very reluctant to try any medication. He works as a support worker at a local homeless hostel and can find this very stressful at times. He has some contact with his mother and older sister, and spends a lot of time with Claire's family. Jack has a number of interests including playing badminton and pool; he also spends a lot of time playing video games.

Claire has recently become very concerned as she feels Jack is withdrawing from her and is spending more and more time playing video games. He has turned down several invites to play pool from a friend and has missed the last two badminton games because he says he was tired. Their GP has suggested a referral to the surgery counsellor but Jack says he is fine, just tired, and doesn't need anyone trying to get into his head. Claire is finding it increasingly difficult to cope with Jack's behaviour and has approached a local carer group for advice.

Questions

- Who are the members of Jack's support network who may have different views and information?

- What support is available in your local area to help Claire in this situation?

Summary

This section of the workbook has considered individual needs and strengths, and how the social system can be drawn upon and worked with to enhance support and promote recovery. It is clear that a person has a wide range of interactions and support mechanisms, and each of these can have an impact upon the individual's well-being. The definition of this capability is:

> *'Working in partnership to gather information to agree health and social care needs in the context of the preferred lifestyle and aspirations of service users their families, carers and friends.'*

Strengths come in many forms and every person has a range of personal, social and spiritual strengths as well as needs. Services have traditionally focused upon treatment and cure and this can be a limiting perspective. Recovery takes many forms and is defined by the individual themself. As such, a wider view of the person within their context, and the role of that context, is needed to ensure that a personalised approach is taken and the principles of social capital, partnership and individual choice and control are all embedded within support systems.

Summary exercise

Write a short summary of what this capability means to you in your context/practice, and then answer the following three questions.

- What have you learnt by completing this section?

- How have you now reached competence in this area?

- What do you need to do to maintain your competence?

References

Allen R, Gilbert P & Onyett S (2009) *Leadership for Personalisation and Social Inclusion in Mental Health*. SCIE, Adult Services Report 27. London: SCIE.

Allott P (2002) Discovering hope for recovery from a British perspective: a review of a selection of recovery literature, implications for practice and systems change. In: S Lime, M McCubbin & B Dallgire (Eds) International Innovations in Community Mental Health (Special Issue). *Canadian Journal of Community Mental Health* **21** (3).

Anthony WA (1993) Recovery from mental illness: the guiding vision of the mental health service system in the 1990s. *Psychosocial Rehabilitation Journal* **16** (4) 11–23.

Bartlett A, Smith G & King M (2009) *The Response of Mental Health Professionals to Clients Seeking Help to Change or Redirect Same-sex Sexual Orientation*. Division of Mental Health, St George's Hospital, University of London/Department of Mental Health Sciences, University College Hospital, University of London.

Beresford P (2002) Thinking about 'mental health': towards a social model. *Journal of Mental Health* **11** (6) 581–584.

Boehnlein JK (2000) *Psychiatry and Religion: The convergence of mind and spirit. Issues in psychiatry*. Arlington, VA: American Psychiatric Press Inc.

Cocker C & Hafford-Letchfield T (2010) Out and proud? Social work's relationship with lesbian and gay equality. *British Journal of Social Work* [online]. Advanced Access published online March 2010. Available at: http://bjsw.oxfordjournals.org/cgi/content/abstract/bcp158v1 (accessed June2010.

CSCI (2008) Putting people first: equality and diversity matters 1. Providing appropriate services for lesbian, gay, bisexual and transgender people. *Social Care Policy and Practice* **7**. London: CSCI.

Davidson L (2008) *Recovery – Concepts and application* [online]. Devon Recovery Group. Available at: www.scmh.org.uk (accessed June 2010).

Department of Health (2007) *An Introduction to Working with Lesbian, Gay and Bisexual People* [online]. London: TSO. Available at: http://www.dh.gov.uk/en/Publicationsandstatistics/Publications/PublicationsPolicyAndGuidance/DH_074255 (accessed June 2010).

Department of Health (2008a) *Carers at the Heart of 21st Century Families and Communities: A caring system on your side, a life of your own*. London: TSO.

Department of Health (2008b) *Putting People First: Transforming adult social care*. London: Department of Health [online] http://www.dh.gov.uk/en/Publicationsandstatistics/Publications/PublicationsPolicyAndGuidance/DH_089665 (accessed June 2010).

Department of Health (2009) *New Horizons: Towards a shared vision for mental health – Consultation*. London: TSO.

Duggan M, Cooper A & Foster J (2002) *Modernising the Social Model in Mental Health: A discussion paper*. London: SPN and TOPPS.

Fish J (2007) *Mental Health Issues within Lesbian, Gay and Bisexual (LGB) Communities*, DH, NHS, Briefing 9. London: TSO.

Fish J (2009) Invisible no more? Including lesbian, gay and bisexual people in social work and social care. *Practice: Social Work in Action* **21** (1) 47–64.

Glendinning C, Hudson B & Means R (2005) Under strain? Exploring the troubled relationship between health and social care. *Public Money and Management* **25** (4) 245–251.

Koenig HG (2005) *Faith and Mental Health: Religious resources for healing*. West Conshohocken, PA: Templeton Press.

MacFarlane L (1998) *Diagnosis Homophobia: The experiences of lesbians, gay men and bisexuals in mental health services* [online]. London: PACE. Available at: http://www.pacehealth.org.uk/publications (accessed June 2010).

Manthorpe J & Bowes A (2010) Age, ethnicity and equalities: synthesising policy and practice messages from two recent studies of elder abuse in the UK. *Social Policy and Society* **9** (2) 255–265.

McCashen W (2005) *The Strengths Approach*. Bendigo: St. Lukes Innovative Resources.

Mental Health Foundation (2006) *The Impact of Spirituality on Mental Health: A review of the literature* [online]. London: Mental Health Foundation. Available at: http://www.rcpsych.ac.uk/pdf/Mental%20Health%20Foundation%20spirituality%20reportx.pdf (accessed June 2010).

National Institute for Mental Health in England (2007) *National Suicide Prevention Strategy for England, Annual report on progress 2006*. London: NIMHE/DH.

National Mental Health Development Unit (2010) *Paths to Personalisation – A whole system, whole life framework*. London: NMHDU/DH.

Owen S & Khalil E (2007) Addressing diversity in mental health care: a review of guidance documents. *International Journal of Nursing Studies* **44** (3) 467–478.

PACE (2008) Project Evaluation: 'Mental Health Advocacy' Project for Advice, Counselling and Education (PACE). London: Kings Fund. Available at: http://www.pacehealth.org.uk/publications

RCP/SCIE (2007) *A Common Purpose: Recovery in future mental health services*. London: SCIE.

Shepherd G, Boardman J & Slade M (2008) *Making Recovery a Reality*. London: Sainsbury Centre for Mental Health.

Sims A & Cook CCH (2009) Spirituality in Psychiatry. In: C Cook, A Powell & A Sims (Eds) *Spirituality and Psychiatry*. London: Royal College of Psychiatry.

Slade M (2009) *100 Ways to Support Recovery: A guide for mental health professionals* [online]. Rethink recovery series volume 1. London: Rethink. Available at: http://www.rethink.org/100ways (accessed June 2010).

Social Exclusion Unit (2003) *Mental Health and Social Exclusion*. TSO: London.

Taylor SE & Brown JD (1988) Illusion and well-being: a social psychological perspective on mental health. *Psychological Bulletin* **103** (2) 193–210.

Turton P, Wright C, White S, Killaspy H & the DEMpBinc Group (2010) Promoting recovery in long-term institutional mental health care: an international Delphi study. *Psychiatric Services* **61** (3) 293–299.

Young SL & Ensing DS (1999) Exploring recovery from the perspective of people with psychiatric disabilities. *Psychiatric Rehabilitation Journal* **22** (3) 219–231.

Section 7: Providing service user-centred care

Negotiating achievable and meaningful goals; primarily from the perspective of service users and their families. Influencing and seeking the means to achieve these goals and clarifying the responsibilities of the people who will provide any help that is needed, including systematically evaluating outcomes and achievements.

Person-centred care is a concept that has received significant emphasis (Robertson *et al*, 2005; Adams & Grieder, 2005; Barker, 2001), and has become more embedded within mental health care over the life of the last National Service Framework (DH, 1999), which is continuing into the New Horizons strategy (DH, 2009a). The recognition that recovery is an individual journey, and hence must focus on the person's hopes, strengths and needs, has become a fundamental aspect of mental health service delivery, and as the personalised approach becomes more embedded, the drive towards meaningful partnership and co-production between service users and worker/service providers will continue to be emphasised as a central component of quality and effective support.

Aims

This section of the workbook focuses on the direct link between person-centred approaches and the personalisation agenda, with specific attention paid to the role of partnership and co-production as the means by which individuals using services can be empowered to exercise choice, control and self-direction. As such, the aims of this section are:

- to place individual goal setting at the centre of the personalised approach
- to explore how person-centred care links into the promotion of mental health recovery
- to explore the role of partnership and co-production as the cornerstone of self-direction, choice and control for individuals experiencing mental distress.

Overview

Personalisation can be seen as an extension of the original concepts used in person-centred care, and as an approach, which focuses upon self-direction and self-determination. From a recovery perspective, the focus on the goals and strengths that are required within this competency assists the individual to define their own pathway and journey.

Six areas of competence are included within this shared capability, these are:

Competence 1:	Work alongside the service user to help them to describe their goals as precisely as possible in a way that is meaningful to them.
Competence 2:	Help the service user to identify and use their strengths to achieve their goals and aspirations.
Competence 3:	Identify the strengths and resources within the service user's wider network which have a role to play in supporting goal achievement.
Competence 4:	Ensure that any goal setting is driven by the needs of the service user.
Competence 5:	Ensure that any goals are achievable and measurable.
Competence 6:	Understand the difference between broader long-term and short-term, more specific goals.

The strengths and resources the person has are often not at the forefront of their thinking at times of distress. It is vital that workers are able to help the individual to identify the positives about their situation and to focus on personal aspirations and aims if they are to fully implement personalised support. For service users and carers, working through this section will help to identify individual goals and provide direction in terms of what can be achieved in the recovery context. These competencies contribute to the individual's choices and control over their situation by promoting independence and highlighting the personal strengths that each individual has.

By working through these competencies the reader will be able to link personalisation, recovery and person-centred planning together to assist the individual to set realistic and meaningful goals.

Competence 1

Work alongside the service user to help them to describe their goals as precisely as possible in a way that is meaningful to them.

Setting personal goals can be a complex task, especially at times when the individual is experiencing distress and anxiety. The symptoms of mental health difficulties often lead to negative thinking and a lack of self-belief and self-esteem, and setting goals within this context can be difficult. However, breaking down hopes and aspirations into small and achievable tasks can also have a positive impact upon the individual's well-being and motivation, increasing confidence and their sense of self-worth, and positively supporting recovery as a consequence (Jacobson & Greenley, 2001; Young & Ensing, 1999; Emmons *et al*, 1998).

Being specific and precise about what it is that the person wants to achieve is important in the goal setting process as it helps to focus on the tasks that need to be undertaken, and also makes the goal more manageable and measureable. This in itself can help the individual to stay motivated about their goals as it makes progress visible and reinforces any achievements that are being made. The specifics of any goals need to be meaningful for the person, and as such, these goals and aims need to be identified by the individual and not imposed by others. Exploring what each aim means can help to ensure that this is the case and it can also help the individual to understand what it is they would like to achieve.

Example

Overall aim: I want to be healthier

In this statement it is important to define what this means to the person – is it that they want to improve their physical or mental health, do they want to be fitter, to lose weight, to have a better diet, or all of these things? Exploring these issues will help to make the goal more specific and will also help the individual to understand what they are aiming for.

Specific goal: I want to take regular exercise and be able to run three miles without discomfort.

Reflection exercise

Identify a personal aspiration that you have and consider what this would be in specific terms. Ask yourself what your overall aim means and break this down into a precise statement about what it is you want to achieve.

Competence 2

Help the service user to identify and use their strengths to achieve their goals and aspirations.

Identifying strengths is a difficult process as at times of distress it is more likely that the person focuses on the negatives and difficulties they are experiencing. Despite these feelings, every individual has strengths that they are able to draw upon, and the strengths approach is something that is consistent with both recovery and the personalisation approach.

The strengths-based approach rests on several principles, these are:

- the focus of the helping process is upon the individual's strengths, interests, abilities and capabilities, not upon their deficits, weaknesses or problems
- all individuals have the capacity to learn, grow and change
- the service user–worker relationship becomes a primary and essential partnership, with the service user viewed as the leader of the helping process
- the local neighbourhood is viewed as a source of potential resources rather than as an obstacle. Natural neighbourhood and community resources should be considered before segregated mental health services.

Ryan & Morgan, 2004; Morgan, 2004

This model supports both the social capital and the choice and control elements of the personalisation approach as well as supporting self-efficacy and contributing to increasing confidence, both of which are central to the recovery model. As such, mental health service users and practitioners need to work together to identify and use the strengths of the individual (Rapp, 1998; Morgan, 2004). Strengths can take different forms, ranging from personal characteristics, preferences, behaviours and experiences, to social networks and support mechanisms that can be drawn upon. The range of strengths that an individual has may help them work towards, and achieve, the goals they have set for themselves, and it is important that these are identified and worked with.

Reflection exercise

Consider the goal you specified for Competence 1.

What are the strengths that you have to help you to achieve the goal?

Consider: preferences and interests, past experience, behaviours and emotional reactions, people who support you, activities that could or do help, community groups, services or organisations you could draw up, family and friends who could input or provide assistance or advice.

Competence 3

Identify the strengths and resources within the service user's wider network which have a role to play in supporting goal achievement.

A range of influences can help or hinder the personal achievement of goals, and it is helpful to identify these. Both people and personal characteristics and behaviours can have an impact, and factors that can help to maintain motivation are important to consider.
While this competence concerns those aspects which support goal achievement, it is also important to be aware of the barriers that need to be overcome – this is part of ensuring that the goal is realistic and achievable for the person and helps to prepare and support them as they work towards their aims. Considering a specific goal as an example, and identifying the possible influences on the achievement of this, is a helpful way to understand this competence and provides a template to work through for application to the practice situation.

Possible strengths	Example goal	Possible barriers
Personal skills and experiences →	To apply for, and secure a job as a support worker with the local mental health services	← Personal skills and experiences
Family and friends →		← Lack of references
Previous work and voluntary work options →		← Financial situation
Support groups and community groups →		← Lack of ongoing support
User-led organisations and peer support →		← Attitudes to mental health
Training and education options and experiences →		← Availability of opportunities

The strengths and resources available to the individual within the wider network can help them to overcome some of the barriers that they may face when working towards their goals.

For example, in the issue set out above it may be that recent references from an employer are not available, however, if the individual is accessing local community groups this may provide them with the references they need to gain employment.

Activity

Using the above template, identify a specific goal and set out the possible strengths, resources and support available to the person, as well as any barriers that impact upon the achievement of the goal.

Questions to be considered:

- Do any of the strengths help to minimise the barriers identified?

- Are other resources needed to support achievement of the goal?

The social capital element of the personalisation approach is key to this competence as it considers the wider networks and community support mechanisms, and encourages thinking beyond the individual and their immediate situation. Community groups, for example, can provide valuable advice and experiences, including social interactions, which would not have otherwise been available to the person.

The personal and social context can have a significant impact on whether a stated goal is achievable (Gollwitzer, 1993; Grant & Dwenck, 2003; Ruehlman & Wolchik, 1988), and considering the wider network provides the opportunity to work through the possibilities and pitfalls associated with achieving any individual goal.

Competence 4

Ensure that any goal setting is driven by the needs of the service user.

The emphasis on self-assessment within the personalisation approach assists in ensuring that the individual's needs and goals are central to the process. However, it should be noted that this is a distinct shift in the way that services have traditionally operated. Within mental health services there is a culture of 'professional knows best', which needs to be continually challenged. Aspects such as risk behaviour, whether this is as a result of substance misuse, vulnerability or perceived possible aggression, continue to be a concern to both the public and service providers (DH, 2009b; Lauber *et al*, 2006; Cass *et al*, 2009), and the culture of risk aversion within the system should not be underestimated if this competence is to be achieved.

As discussed elsewhere in this workbook, person-centred planning and support has helped to place the service user in the central position, and aspects of personalisation such as self-assessment, personal budgets and a wider choice of support packages and services is helping to shift the attitudes within services. However, it is still common for goals to be heavily influenced by what workers feel is required, and these need to be identified and challenged. The impact of the legal sanctions that can be used within the mental health system and the impact of coercive treatment will remain a reality, and as such, goal setting needs to acknowledge these influences and ensure that goals are negotiated and agreed, and are not simply imposed in the individual's 'best interests' (DH, 2007a; DH, 2007b; Langan & Lindow, 2004; Bogg, 2008).

A holistic view of an individual's life needs to be considered within the initial assessment and subsequent goal planning process, and personalisation supports this aim as it considers the social context of a person, and includes the range of relationships and networks that an individual may have or desire (Carr, 2008; Brewis, 2007).

The development and implementation of self-assessment models varies across local authority areas, a number of examples are available via the Department of Health Care networks personalisation portal at www.dhcarenetworks.org.uk/personalisation/index.cfm. The common themes across those areas which have developed a self-assessment process, and indeed within the model tools, is the widespread of areas that are considered, and the inclusion of lifestyle, activity, vocation and relationship issues as well as more traditional personal and social care needs. Goal setting within mental health support needs to ensure that these areas are considered, and that the recovery areas the individual identifies are encompassed within the planning processes.

Case study exercise

Read the following case study and identify possible goals that are consistent with the presenting needs of Elaine.

Elaine has been using mental health services for the last few years and has a diagnosis of bipolar disorder. She is in her early 30s and has recently ended a relationship with a local man (who she has been friends with for several years) because she felt he didn't understand the difficulties she was having and kept telling her to 'pull herself together'. Elaine's family all live quite a distance away and while she has phone contact with them, she does not visit very often as she has no transport.

Elaine has been unemployed since she lost her job following her initial admission into mental health services, and has taken several distance learning courses since then as she says she needs to focus on something to keep her mind active, but doesn't feel able to join local groups on her own. Elaine's work experience is largely in administration and office management work and she does not want to return to this. She also has a degree in business and administration. She says that she would like to go into adult education teaching or something similar but feels she isn't qualified or confident enough.

Over the last few years Elaine has had difficulties in taking part in activities, she says this has meant that she doesn't exercise as much as she'd like to, that she feels self-conscious and anxious when meeting new people. She used to enjoy creative writing and painting but has not done these for some time – she says she feels lonely and bored a lot of the time.

Competence 5

Ensure that any goals are achievable and measurable.

Any goals that are set by the person need to be both realistic and meaningful, it is very easy to fall into the trap of vague statements relating to hopes for the future, however, these are not helpful and run the risk of setting the person up to fail from the outset. Setting out a goal that is measurable can help the individual to feel that they are making progress and enhance their motivation (Locke,1996; Latham & Locke, 1991), which in times of distress is a valuable reinforcement of the person's hope that recovery is possible for them (Siegert & Taylor, 2004; Stineman *et al*, 2008).

SMART goal setting is a tool that is well known within organisational psychology and performance, and can be applied to mental health recovery to ensure that aims are achievable and can easily be measured and monitored on a regular basis. The principles of SMART goal setting within care planning are not a new concept, and a great deal of research has been carried out in relation to its effectiveness in rehabilitation programmes for a variety of conditions (Playford *et al*, 2000; Stineman *et al*, 2008; Webb & Glueckauf, 1994; Siegert *et al*, 2004; Mueser *et al*, 2002).

Ensuring that a goal is SMART means that it needs to be:

S – Specific: the goal describes the action that the individual will take.

M – Measurable: the goal has a defined outcome and milestones that indicate whether the goal is being achieved.

A – Achievable: the goal is something that the individual is able to achieve within their capabilities and with the resources available to them.

R – Realistic: the goal is a real possibility for the individual.

T – Time-bound: there is an identified timescale for achieving the goal that can be measured.

Being specific is important as it makes the goal meaningful and provides a clear focus. For example, stating that the person wants to attend college is a positive aspiration but as a goal it does not provide a focus, whereas stating that the person will enrol onto a diploma course in business and administration at a specific college in September 2011, allows the individual to take certain clear steps and measure their successes towards that goal.

Exercise

From the following goal statements identify which goals are SMART, and change those which are not into SMART goal statements.

1. I want to travel the world.
2. I will apply for the training scholarship that was advertised in the paper last Thursday by the closing date.
3. I want to start a new job by the end of the year.
4. I will ring my parents once a week from next Tuesday.
5. I want to stop smoking.

6. I will go to the gym twice a week for at least 30 minutes, starting in January.
7. I want to go on holiday to Spain in May.
8. I will make new friends.

In setting measurable and achievable goals, a number of things – which have been discussed within the other competencies within this section – need to be considered. These include: what steps need to be taken to reach the goal? Is the goal realistic for the person at the current time? What are the obstacles to reaching the goal? What resources (including people and other supports) can help to achieve the goal? For each goal it is helpful for the person to set out the steps they will take, this also helps to make it a measurable task and can reinforce progress along the way which helps to keep motivated and focused on the aim.

Example

Goal: To complete a college course in catering by 2012.

Possible steps/milestones

- Ring the college and request an application form by July 2010
- Fill in the required form by August 2010
- Return it to the college by August 2010
- Attend the interview for the course intake in September 2010
- Attend registration for the course and collect the timetable in September 2010
- Attend the required classes from September 2010

Competence 6

Understand the difference between broader long-term and short-term, more specific goals.

While we all have long-term aspirations, things that we would like to do with our lives, time or careers, there needs to be an awareness of what constitutes long-term hopes and what are specific goals in order to be able to set out steps that may be taken and retain focus on what we are trying to achieve. Long-term goals are usually larger tasks that will be achieved over a period of time – this can be several months, years, or indeed a lifetime, whereas short-term goals are usually more specific and have a shorter timescale that is tangible to the individual – usually days or weeks, with identified milestones that support motivation and focus on the aim (Locke, 1996; Latham & Locke, 1991; Berry & West, 1993).

The longer-term goals are often those that are most meaningful to us, being hopes and dreams for our personal futures. However, the extended timescales and the wider definitions of these goals mean that it can be difficult to remain focused and motivated, or to measure the progress that is being made at any point in time.

Example

I want to get married and have children.

For a single person this is a significant change and involves a number of steps including meeting possible partners. It is difficult to measure this goal and can lead to an over emphasis on the outcome rather than the process.

Short-term goals do need to be in line with the longer-term plan but are often more useful within the mental health and personalisation context as they enable the wider aims to be broken down into more manageable pieces, which reinforce personal achievement and make the task feel more accessible, especially during periods of distress when the larger context can be overwhelming for the individual.

Example

I would like to go on a date in the next six weeks.

This goal is more achievable in the immediate term than getting married and having children, and could involve accessing a range of activities including singles events, dating sites and other social options as the first step towards the longer-term aim of having a family.

Linking long-term and short-term goals is an important factor to consider as there needs to be a connection between what the person ultimately wants to achieve and the efforts they are making in the immediate future. This helps to reinforce the goals at each stage and assists in the achievement of the goals themselves (Brunstein, 1993; Locke, 1996; Locke & Latham, 1990).

Within a personalised approach the aim is for the individual to have choice and control over their own situation, and as such, it is important that they set their own long-term and short-term options. The competence within this area is to identify the differences between the bigger and longer-term aims, and the specific short-term actions that will support them to reach their desired state.

Exercise

- Identify which of the following goals are long-term and which are short-term.
- Each long-term goal has a short-term goal that will support it. Identify the links between the goals.

To be healthy and slimmer	To be successful in my career
To get a degree	To submit my recent article for publication
To buy the local paper on job day	To sail around the world
To become a successful writer	To attend the gym twice a week
To apply for an advertised promotion	To get a job
To send for the university prospectus	To identify the countries I would like to visit

Summary

The overall capability that has been considered within this section is providing service user-centred care, which means:

'*Negotiating achievable and meaningful goals; primarily from the perspective of service users and their families. Influencing and seeking the means to achieve these goals and clarifying the responsibilities of the people who will provide any help that is needed, including systematically evaluating outcomes and achievements.*'

These competencies have presented and explored the role of goal setting within the planning processes for individuals, and highlighted the need to identify specific aims and draw upon the strengths of the individual to achieve the goals they have set for themselves. These areas are important within both personalisation and the recovery approach, and individuals need to be supported to highlight and explore their personal aspirations if they are to be independent and in control of their own circumstances.

Summary exercise

Write a short summary of what this capability means to you in your context/practice, and then answer the following three questions.

- What have you learnt by completing this section?

- How have you now reached competence in this area?

- What do you need to do to maintain your competence?

References

Adams N & Grieder DM (2005) *Treatment Planning for Person-Centred Care: The road to mental health and addiction recovery*. London: Elsevier Press.

Barker P (2001) The tidal model: developing a person-centred approach to psychiatric and mental health nursing. *Perspectives in Psychiatric Care* **37** (3) 79–87.

Berry JM & West RL (1993) Cognitive self-efficacy in relation to personal mastery and goal setting across the lifespan. In ME Lachman (Ed) *Planning and Control Processes Across the Life Span*. Hove: Lawrence Eribaum Associates Ltd.

Bogg D (2008) The Bigger Picture: Perceived Risk is a Barrier to User-led provision. *Mental Health Today*, September 2008, 19.

Brewis R (2007) *A Voice and A Choice: Self directed support for people with mental health problems* [online]. Available at: http://www.dhcarenetworks.org.uk/_library/Resources/Personalisation/Personalisation_advice/A_Voice_and_Choice_Sept_07_Rita_Brewis_IC.pdf (accessed June 2010).

Brunstein JC (1993) Personal goals and subjective well-being: a longitudinal study. *Journal of Personality & Social Psychology* **65** (5) 1061–1070.

Carr S (2008) *Personalisation: A Rough Guide*. Adult Services Report 20. London: SCIE.

Cass E, Robbins D & Richardson A (2009) Dignity in Care Within Mental Health: Tackling stigma. Guide 15, 3rd update. London: SCIE.

Department of Health (1999) *National Service Framework for Mental Health*. London: TSO.

Department of Health (2007a) *Best Practice in Managing Risk: Principles and evidence for best practice in the assessment and management of risk to self and others in mental health services*. London: TSO.

Department of Health (2007b) *Independence, Choice and Risk: A guide to best practice in supported decision making*. London: TSO.

Department of Health (2009a) *New Horizons: Towards a Shared Vision for Mental Health – Consultation*. London: TSO.

Department of Health (2009b) *Attitudes to Mental Illness research report 2009*. Available at: http://www.dh.gov.uk/en/Publicationsandstatistics/PublishedSurvey/ListOfSurveySince1990/Surveylistmentalhealth/index.htm

Emmons RA, Colby PM & Kaiser HA (1998) When losses lead to gains: personal goals and the recovery of meaning. In IB Wiener (Ed) *The Human Quest for Meaning: A handbook of psychological research and clinical applications*. London: Routledge.

Gollwitzer PM (1993) Goal achievement: the role of intentions. *European Review of Social Psychology* **4** 141–185.

Grant H & Dweck, CS (2003) Clarifying Achievement Goals and Their Impact. *Journal of Personality & Social Psychology* **85** (3) 541–553.

Jacobson N & Greenley D (2001) What is recovery? A conceptual model and explication. *Psychiatric Services* **52** 482–485.

Langan J & Lindow V (2004) *Mental health service users and their involvement in risk assessment and management* [online]. York: Joseph Rowntree Foundation. Available at: http://www.jrf.org.uk/publications/mental-health-service-users-and-their-involvement-risk-assessment-and-management (accessed June 2010).

Latham GP & Locke EA (1991) Self-regulation through goal setting. *Organizational Behaviour and Human Decision Making Processes* **50** (2) 212–247.

Lauber C, Nordt C, Braunschweig C & Rossler W (2006) Do mental health professionals stigmatise their patients? *Acta Psychiatrica Scandinavica* **113** (s429) 51–59.

Locke EA (1996) Motivation through Conscious Goal Setting. *Applied & Preventative Psychology* **5** (2) 117–124.

Locke EA & Latham GP (1990) *A Theory of Goal Setting and Task Performance*. New Jersey: Prentice Hall.

Morgan S (2004) Strengths Based Practice. *Open Mind*, March/April 2004, 126–127.

Mueser KT, Corrigan PW, Hilton DW, Tanzman B, Schuab A, Ginderich S, Essock SM, Tarrier N, Morey B, Vogel-Scibilia S & Herx MI (2002) Illness management and recovery: a review of the research. *Psychiatric Services* **53** 1272–1284.

Playford ED, Dawson L, Limbert V, Smith M, Ward CD & Wells R (2000) Goal-setting in rehabilitation: report of a workshop to explore professionals' perceptions of goal-setting. *Clinical Rehabilitation* **14** (5) 491–496.

Rapp C (1998) *The Strengths Model: Case management with people suffering from severe and persistent mental illness*. New York: Oxford University Press.

Robertson J, Emerson E, Hatton C, Elliott J, McIntosh B, Swift P, Krinjen-Kemp E, Towers C, Romeo R, Knapp M, Sanderson H, Routledge M, Oakes P & Joyce T (2005) *The Impact of Person Centred Planning*. Lancaster: Institute for Health Research, Lancaster University.

Ruehlman LS & Wolchik SA (1988) Personal Goals and Interpersonal Support and Hindrance as Factors in Psychological Distress and Well-Being. *Journal of Personality and Social Psychology* **55** (2) 293–301.

Ryan P & Morgan S (2004) *Assertive Outreach: A strengths approach to policy and practice*. Edinburgh: Churchill Livingstone.

Siegert RJ & Taylor WJ (2004) Theoretical aspects of goal setting and motivation in rehabilitation. *Disability & Rehabilitation* **26** (1) 1–8.

Siegert RJ, McPherson KM & Taylor W (2004) Towards a cognitive-affective model of goal setting in rehabilitation: is self-regulation theory a key step? *Disability & Rehabilitation* **26** (20) 1175–1183.

Stineman MG, Kurz AE, Kelleher D & Kennedy BL (2008) The patient's view of recovery: An emerging tool for empowerment through self-knowledge. *Disability & Rehabilitation* **30** (9) 679–68.

Webb PM & Glueckauf RL (1994) The effects of direct involvement in goal setting on rehabilitation outcome for persons with traumatic brain injuries. *Rehabilitation Psychology* **39** (3) 179–188.

Young SL & Ensing D (1999) Exploring recovery from the perspective of people with psychiatric disabilities. *Psychiatric Rehabilitation Journal* **22** (3) 219–232.

Section 8: Making a difference

Facilitating access to and delivering the best quality, evidence-based, values-based health and social care interventions to meet the needs and aspirations of service users and their families and carers.

Quality and evidence-based services have been the focus of the majority of mental health policies and strategies for a number of years and recent reviews and publications continue that focus. The National Service Framework (DH, 1999) started the drive towards evidence-based developments by rating available evidence on a five-point scale according to how reliable the findings were. The New Horizons strategy (DH, 2009) continues this drive, stating:

'Service improvements will need to be self-financing, soundly evidence-based, and clearly related to local commissioning intentions.' (p10)

There is a range of research and evidence available, which mental health support and treatment is based on, and this comes from medical, psychological, social care and survivor studies and reviews. Bodies such as the National Institute of Clinical Excellence (NICE), the Social Care Institute for Excellence (SCIE), and the National Mental Health Development Unit (NMHDU), as well as other Department of Health and academic groups, all regularly publish findings and guidance to inform practices across the mental health system. As such, those involved in mental health support services need to be aware of the evidence-base, that is underpinning policy and driving change, to inform the assessment, risk management, care and support planning processes.

Aims

Personalisation and recovery provide a range of outcomes that can be used to make sure support is tailored to the individual, and this section makes the link between best practice, recovery and personalisation in mental health settings. The overall aims of the section are:

- to link best practice, personalisation and recovery in mental health
- to provide an overview of the evidence and value-base of a personalised approach
- to provide a direct link between best practice and individual needs, strengths, and aspirations.

Overview

The needs of individuals are unique and diverse, and workers and services need to be able to assess and plan, together with the service user, to understand the issues and work towards making changes. Making a difference in someone's life means being able to work from their understanding of the situation and towards the goals they have set for themselves, a person-centred, strength based approach.

Six areas of competence are included within this shared capability, these are:

Competence 1:	Understand the impact of any particular problem on the life of the service user and their family and friends.
Competence 2:	Understand the notions of evidence-based and values-based 'best practice' as enshrined in NICE guidance and psychosocial interventions training etc.
Competence 3:	Have the ability to design, or contribute to the design of a programme of care based on 'best practice' or the best available evidence.
Competence 4:	Understand the role that they may play in a programme of care based on 'best practice'.
Competence 5:	Understand the role that others may play in such a programme.
Competence 6:	Communicate with all, including service users and carers, who have a part to play in a programme of care.

There is a range best practice information and guidance available for workers and service users to draw upon to inform the care and support planning process, and understanding the person's individual circumstances is the basis on which all interventions should focus. The term care and support plan is used throughout this section, there are differences in how this terminology is used and in some cases the term support plan is used to mean just the plan that details how social care resource allocation is to be used. In this section care and support plan means a plan that includes both the interventions and treatment that an individual may have and also any purchased care – an integrated planning process is used here because it reflects the joined up nature of mental health services.

There are some tensions that exist between evidence and individual preference and individuals need to be aware of these if they are to consider evidence-based practice within the personalisation of mental health. First, it is worth remembering that research evidence is not a complete science; there are contexts and limitations that influence the findings. Any research that is carried out is usually from the perspective of the researcher, which creates a bias towards one outcome or another. Additionally, there is only evidence of methods that have been researched. This does not mean that other approaches would not work but rather that other approaches have not yet been investigated.

One further issue of note here is that there may be a difference between what a service user feels is working and what a carer or other family member or friend feels works. This can be difficult and at times creates conflict and the worker will need to ensure that all views are considered and any conflicts are managed carefully.

There are some principles that need to guide people as they consider the evidence base within mental health settings, these are as follows.

- An awareness that much 'evidence' in mental health is produced from research perspectives that do not necessarily embrace current principles of recovery and independent living.

- Evidence may be as much about effectiveness in general terms rather than for any particular person. This is known as a utilitarian approach, which means it aims to help as many people as possible rather than be tailored to individual needs.
- Evidence that something has beneficial effects does not mean there are not other equally beneficial (and possibly totally different) options that have not been researched.
- Evidence that exists at present exists for those things that people have chosen to investigate, which itself has been determined to a large extent by traditional and professional notions of research and 'suitability'.
- The boundary of self-determination needs to be clearly understood in order that people are not obliged to accept a treatment or intervention that is considered to be effective but which they do not want, unless legally obliged to do so.
- The 'evidence' of what a person believes and/or finds works best for them is a crucial part of any decision that is truly based on all available evidence. This is not from a traditional evidence base, but rather focuses on the individual's lived experience.
- The formal evidence base is there to guide practitioners and service providers as to what they should offer/recommend to people.
- People creating their own strategies to manage their mental health can only create evidence of effectiveness by being allowed to try.

Workers and service users need to bear these principles in mind throughout this section and within the field of evidence-based practice generally. Personalisation encourages new approaches and emphasises the experience of the individual. These areas have not been researched to a great extent to date, however, and lived experience is something that needs serious exploration if we are to do more than just rebrand the more traditional approaches.

Competence 1

Understand the impact of any particular problem on the life of the service user and their family and friends.

Both the recovery approach and the personalisation approach are focused upon the individual and their experience, and as such, individual strengths and problems need to be explored and understood to be able to tailor care and support to the specific needs of the person. Evidence shows that mental health issues are widespread and are influenced by a number of factors, including social, psychological and health-based issues (Frese *et al*, 2001; Kelly & Gamble, 2005; RCP/SCIE, 2007).

The recovery approach presented in section 5 showed that many areas of a person's life, including employment, finances and personal relationships can have a bearing on mental health difficulties. As a result, there needs to be a full consideration of the person's context within the assessment process to ensure that all areas that may be relevant are identified. A range of tools are available to support holistic assessments, however, the emphasis on self-direction and self-assessment is becoming more common in the social care context, and while the assessment cannot be wholly self-assessed (ADASS, 2009) because of the legal duty on councils to assess needs, there is still an emphasis on person-led assessment processes. Mental health providers are struggling with the principle of person-led assessment due to the issues of risk management and protection, and it seems that while self-assessment is the aim, this is largely carried out alongside professional assessment rather than as a stand-alone activity.

The new mental health strategy *New Horizons* (DH, 2009) emphasises outcomes as the key focus for support processes, and the recovery star (MacKeith & Burns, 2008) is identified as the tool for assessment of needs and outcomes of adults of working age. A self-rated scale, which indentifies the issues in a person's life in a range of areas, assists with the care and support planning and provides a baseline from which a person can measure their own progress.

Recovery star tool

Scale: 1–10 rating, with 1 being a serious problem and 10 indicating self-reliance

Domains:

Managing mental health	Self-care
Living skills	Social networks
Work	Relationships
Addictive behaviour	Responsibilities
Identity and self-esteem	Trust and hope

It should be noted that other tools are available, however, the guidance from the Department of Health (DH, 2009) recommends the use of the star in mental health services.

Risk management and professional approaches appear to be the barriers to self-assessment in mental health settings and professional anxiety about risk is still a common issue. The recovery star (and other holistic assessment tools) can be a good starting point for a partnership between service user and worker and there is evidence that suggests that a shared responsibility for risk assessment and management can have positive outcomes for individuals (DH, 2007; Morgan, 2000; Needham & Carr, 2009; SCIE, 2009). Whatever tools are used by services, there is a need to ensure that the person's whole situation is considered and a shared understanding of the issues and what impact they have on the person's mental health. From this starting point, service users and workers will be able to work together within care and support planning and ensure that services are tailored to the individual's needs and strengths.

Case study exercise

David is a 32-year-old man who has recently separated from his wife. He has two children both under five years old, who live with their mother. David has weekend contact, and has moved into a flat in the local area. David has been in contact with mental health services recently as he has been experiencing depression since his separation and is also drinking more than normal. He is very low, and does not want to do anything. His mother has been visiting every few days but says that he rarely leaves his bedroom. David is unemployed and says he 'has nothing worth getting up for and so he'll stay here'; he does make short trips to the off-licence and then returns to his bedroom. He is not eating properly and has not bathed for some time. David talks to a worker from the team and says that he would like things to be different and he is tired of feeling bad, but he doesn't know what to do to make things better and he has no energy to try anything new.

Questions

- Using the recovery star domains, what areas are relevant to David's care, and what do you think he would score himself?

Competence 2

Understand the notions of evidence-based and values-based 'best practice' as enshrined in NICE guidance and psychosocial interventions training etc.

While evidence-based and values-based practice are often linked within guidance, there are key differences in the two approaches, and it is helpful to define each of these terms.

- Evidence-based practice means that the treatment that is used has some form of scientific and objective basis to support its use. This can be via research, clinical trials or other consultation and study methods that show a clear outcome for the service user as a result of a particular intervention.
- Values-based practice means that practice takes account of the values, views and perspectives of the person (and their support network), and that the worker pays attention to their own values to make sure decisions are in the best interests of the person, and not unduly influenced by their presumptions and beliefs. This is a far more subjective approach, which has the person central to any practice.

These definitions are not definitive, and there are variations of what is meant by each term, however, for ease of use the statements set out here are used for this section of the workbook.

Mental health services are required to demonstrate evidence and values within their approaches, and there is a range of resources that can be accessed to support workers in this aim. Organisations such as the National Institute for Clinical Excellence (NICE) and the Social Care Institute for Excellence (SCIE) provide a range of briefings, research summaries and best practice guidance, and it is an essential part of practice to be aware of the resources available and the recommended ways of working. Evidence exists for each condition and is based on different criteria. It would be impossible to present all of the information here, however, to have competence in this area workers need to be aware of the following resources all of which provide a range of information on the evidence-base for mental health interventions. It is important to remember when considering these resources that research is not an objective activity and there is a need to remain critical of findings. NICE evidence, for example, does not focus on service user views, and as such, the personalisation focus is not fully accounted for within the recommendations made.

As mental health spans health and social care it needs to be noted that the research methods from each of these areas is very different, and what counts as valid in each field can vary. Clinical trials, for example, are prominent in health research, with NICE and other evidence review bodies placing emphasis on this method over others. Whereas in social care terms, the perspective of users and carers has a much greater emphasis, and qualitative evidence, which is based on views and opinions, is considered to have greater validity (Tew *et al*, 2006; Pawson *et al*, 2003). The argument about which approach is most appropriate to mental health cannot be analysed in any depth here, however, those involved in the field and who are considering evidence-based practice need to remain aware of such issues. The key is to ensure they take a critical view and respond to the individual's wishes and preferences of what works for them as the basis for a personalised approach to evidence-based practice.

General mental health evidence resources

Social Care Institute for Excellence (SCIE) http://www.scie.org.uk
NHS Evidence Library Mental Health http://www.library.nhs.uk/mentalhealth/
National Institute of Clinical Excellence (NICE) http://www.nice.org.uk/guidance/
Evidence-based mental health journal http://ebmh.bmj.com/
The Centre for Evidence-based mental health http://cebmh.warne.ox.ac.uk/cebmh/

For personalisation the evidence base is partial, and still being developed, however, there is a great deal of research available that supports inclusive and person-centred approaches and which indicates that the more control an individual has over their situation the better the outcomes. As noted at the outset of this section, just because there is not a research base on which to draw does not mean that interventions may not be effective for the individual and workers need to be aware of the whole range of options and possible creative approaches that may help to support the individual's recovery.

A review of the evidence for personalisation in mental health was conducted by MIND (2009); this concluded that personalisation follows the independent living philosophy. The evidence for independent living is quite well developed, and there has been much research carried out which shows that independent living improves the outcomes for individuals and contributes to their recovery (Spandler & Vick, 2006; Brewis, 2007; Beresford & Wallcroft, 1997; Bond *et al*, 2004; Crane-Ross *et al*, 2000). Studies on direct payments and individual budgets support the overall direction, and for both users and carers these show improved quality of life as a result of receiving budgets or direct payments, and being able to control and adapt their own support packages to meet individual needs (DH, 2003; Stainton & Boyce, 2004; Glendinning *et al*, 2008; Manthorpe *et al*, 2008). The evidence base for personalisation will continue to develop as the implementation of the programme progresses, however, there are many resources available to inform practice, and some of these are listed below.

Resources for personalisation evidence

NMHDU Pathways to Personalisation
http://www.nmhdu.org.uk/our-work/personalisation-in-mental-health-emerging-programme/paths-to-personalisation/

DH Care Networks Personalisation
http://www.dhcarenetworks.org.uk/personalisation/index.cfm

DH Personalisation Pages
http://www.dh.gov.uk/en/SocialCare/Socialcarereform/Personalisation/index.htm

SCIE Personalisation Resources
http://www.scie.org.uk/adults/personalisation.asp

The Norah Fry Centre
http://www.bristol.ac.uk/norahfry/resources/online/#personalisation

Community Care Personalisation Pages
http://www.communitycare.co.uk/blogs/progress-on-personalisation/

Competence 3

Have the ability to design, or contribute to the design of, a programme of care based on 'best practice' or the best available evidence.

Linking evidence and theory to practice is a skill that all professionally qualified workers will have received some training in. However, the level of capability in this area depends on profession and level of training received. In any event, workers need to be aware of where and how the evidence is collected, and how it applies to their environment. Keeping up to date with developments in the field is a task that can be achieved by reading trade magazines and professional journals, completing training, supervision and peer discussions among other methods, and it is a requirement of all staff to maintain their knowledge. In addition to maintaining knowledge on treatment options and evidence-based practice, workers also need to have a thorough understanding of the locality in which they work and the resources available to be drawn upon in the care and support planning processes.

The assessment is the information that informs the care and support plan and identifies what should be included. Whether the assessment is based on self-assessment or professional assessment, the person's life will have been considered and their needs highlighted and these are the foundation for any plan. The premise is that the evidence base provides the guidance for which interventions show the best outcomes for the needs that have been identified. For example, in a case where the person has schizophrenia and struggles to cope with family relationships it may be that family work is the best option to improve the situation. This conclusion is based on research evidence of the effectiveness of that approach within similar circumstances (NICE, 2010; Addington & Burnett, 2009).

Case study exercise

Sharon is 27 and lives with her parents. She has one sister who lives nearby. She has very few friends and finds socialising with others very difficult. She gets anxious around groups and thinks that people don't like her, which means she spends a lot of time at home on her own. She would like to make friends and meet someone to have a relationship with but says she '*is scared to try*'.

Sharon has a diagnosis of bipolar disorder; she has contact with the local community mental health team and sees a CPN once a fortnight. Sharon takes regular medication, which she says '*slows her down*' and she has problems getting herself motivated to do things. She has recently been having a lot of arguments with her parents who think she needs to get out of the house more often. She feels that they are very critical and don't understand how she feels and this is making the home situation very tense. Both Sharon and her parents are upset about this and want to try and make things better.

Sharon's parents have recently starting going to a carer's group once a week and say this is helping them to cope with Sharon's difficulties.

Sharon has some interests and particularly enjoys painting. She has seen a night class at the local community centre but is worried about going on her own and does not have the equipment she would need and she cannot afford the £50 it would cost. Her sister has volunteered to go with her to the first few classes.

Sharon says her main concerns are around the problems she is having at home and she is feeling lonely and bored and wants to do her painting class.

Activity

Draw up an initial care and support plan for Sharon and consider the following questions.

- What are her needs?
- What are her goals?
- How will the plan support her needs and goals?
- Who will provide each part of the plan?
- Identify any areas which could be addressed with a personal budget or direct payment.

The definition of best practice can be problematic, with perspective and subjectivity causing differences in what is considered 'best'. The outcomes that evidence is based upon can vary, and there needs to be questions asked in terms of how the best outcomes have been defined, who has defined them, is the research or evidence conclusive, and who has input into the process – service users, carers, practitioners? The values that evidence is based upon is usually targeted towards improving the mental health condition. However, as discussed in other sections of this workbook, the condition itself is only a small part of the individual's experience, and the wider context and implications have a direct impact on the person's well-being as well (Tew *et al*, 2006; Pawson *et al*, 2003). In order to apply the principles of best practice and best outcomes, they need to be negotiated with the individual – what is the outcome they desire? A critical view of evidence and what is recommended needs to be maintained.

Competence 4

Understand the role that they may play in a programme of care based on 'best practice'.

It is important to understand the role that each person plays in an individual's care and support plant. There is a wide range of roles in the delivery of mental health services. Under the Care Programme Approach (CPA) the care co-ordinator is responsible for planning and co-ordinating services (DH, 2008) and holds the responsibility, on behalf of the service, for making sure the support that is agreed is delivered to the person.

> *'The care co-ordinator should have the authority to co-ordinate the delivery of the care plan and ensure that this is respected by all those involved in delivering it.'* (DH, 2008, p36)

The role is to have oversight of the whole plan and make sure that everyone involved is providing what they agreed, but it is not necessary to directly provide the services. Community services and groups, informal support networks, other public services and the person themselves may all be involved in making sure the plan happens. The care co-ordinator is the central point of contact and will make sure reviews take place and information is shared where needed.

The revised CPA practice guide makes direct links with the personalisation of mental health, and the care co-ordinator role includes care management and providing access to personal budgets and direct payments, where appropriate. This means that all workers, regardless of profession, who take the care co-ordinator role, need to have a good knowledge of personalisation and what is available for service users to design their own support packages.

Many other services and individuals may be involved in providing support for the person, and whether taking the role of care co-ordinator or not, everyone needs to understand what role they are playing if they are to provide the support the individual needs.

Reflection points

- Do you know how to access social care packages?
- Do you know what a direct payment or personal budget can be used for in your area and what the eligibility criteria are?

Competence 5

Understand the role that others may play in such a programme.

Considering the variety of needs in a person's life, there may be whole range of people or services involved in the plan. Personalisation encourages partnership and co-production between everyone who may play a role in providing support. Therefore, it is important to be aware of the roles of others.

Co-production means working with people as equal partners in the care and support process, this is a change from previous practice and emphasises service user choice and control in shaping and developing the support they need. A briefing published by SCIE in 2009 stated that co-production was used to refer to:

> *'...active input by the people who use services, as well as – or instead of – those who have traditionally provided them ... It emphasises that the people who use services have assets which can help to improve those services, rather than simply needs which must be met.'* (Needham & Carr, 2009)

This partnership between service user and service can also be extended to include carers, other friends or family members who are involved, as well as other groups and organisations. The person has control over their plan and so can specify who should be included or what other support services they may need.

With such variety in who may have a role in the person's support it is important that each person is aware of what they, and others, are responsible for providing. While the care co-ordinator role will help to bring different players together, understanding the whole picture can help to make sure that support is joined-up and tailored to the individual's needs and strengths. Either over-dependence or gaps in support can be a problem for the person with mental health needs, and each person or service should have a distinct role in supporting the individual and promoting their recovery.

Case study exercise

Gareth is a 34-year-old man who lives in a supported flat. He has a support worker, Chris, who he sees twice a week for help with the upkeep of his flat and someone from the housing association visits Gareth in the flat once a month. Gareth is Jewish and goes to synagogue every week; he also likes to spend time talking with the Rabbi.

Gareth's father died a year ago, his mother lives in the next town and he usually sees her once every two weeks when he catches the train to visit.

He has been seen by the mental health team for a few years and sees a social worker, Julie, who he has a good relationship with. He also sees a psychiatrist every now and again.

Gareth wants to get a job and is referred to the local employment service for some help. He also feels quite lonely and would like the chance to meet other people. He has seen some groups that he would like to join but is nervous about this and can't afford transport costs.

Activity

Draw up a plan for Gareth.
Who are the people or services involved in the plan?
What are the roles and responsibilities for each person or service?

Competence 6

Communicate with all, including service users and carers, who have a part to play in a programme of care.

A personalised care and support plan should include the individual themself and their informal support network where they are involved in the programme. Therefore, good communication is needed to make sure there is a consistent approach. Information sharing can be a difficult subject to negotiate, with services concentrating on their own duty of confidentiality. Often the best way to deal with this issue is with the full involvement of the service user, identifying who needs the information and who the individual wants information to be shared with. It is important to make sure that it is clear who needs to be involved in communications.

Communication skills are an important aspect of this competence as it may be that the people involved need different types of information or need it to be given in different ways. One of the key elements in the equality and diversity agenda is making sure that information is accessible for people, and this needs to be applied to information sharing between the people and services involved in the care and support plan. This can involve translating information into different languages, not using jargon, and checking back with individuals that they have understood the agreements and why certain decisions have been made.

Case study exercise

Aadi is a young Indian man who moved to England with his parents as a small child. He has been experiencing paranoia and hearing voices and has been referred to the early intervention in psychosis team by his GP.

He lives with his parents and three brothers. His mother does not speak fluent English but is very supportive and wants to be involved with Aadi's support. The family are asking for information, they want to help but are confused and scared about what is happening to Aadi.

Aadi attends the local college and has a support worker who helps him with his course work; he has dyslexia and has been having attention difficulties but has been enjoying his course and wants to finish it. He also plays five-a-side football with his local pub team and the coach of the team has expressed concerns about Aadi's behaviour, which he says has been erratic.

Questions

- How would you communicate with each of the people involved in Aadi's support network?

- What type of information would you provide to each person involved?

Summary

This capability has considered the role of evidence-based practice in mental health services, and some of the roles that individuals and services play in supporting the person. Care and supporting planning is the way in which services are tailored to meet individual needs, and the partnership between service users and services are central to this process to maximise choice and control and promote recovery.

The overall capability that has been explored is 'making a difference', which means:

Facilitating access to and delivering the best quality, evidence-based, values-based health and social care interventions to meet the needs and aspirations of service users and their families and carers.

The evidence base for personalisation in mental health will continue to develop and those involved in providing support need to make sure they stay up to date with current evidence in order to provide the best support they can for the individual. The exploration of the living experience of individuals is an area that needs to be further developed, as highlighted at the beginning of this section. It must be noted that just because evidence does not yet exist, it does not mean that the approach or intervention is not effective. Each individual's experience of recovery, personalisation and what works for them, is equally valid and in a context of a partial and limited evidence base, tailoring support to individual needs remains the central concern.

Summary exercise

Write a short summary of what this capability means to you in your context/practice, and then answer the following three questions.

- What have you learnt by completing this section?

- How have you now reached competence in this area?

- What do you need to do to maintain your competence?

References

ADASS (2009) *Personalisation and the Law: Implementing Putting People First in the current legal framework*. London: ADASS.

Addington J & Burnett P (2009) Working with families in the early stages of psychosis. In: JFM Gleeson & McGorry PD (Eds) *Psychological Interventions in Early Psychosis: A treatment handbook*. West Sussex: John Wiley & Sons Ltd.

Beresford P & Wallcraft J (1997) Psychiatric system survivors and emancipatory research: issues, overlaps and differences. In: C Barnes & G Mercer (Eds) *Doing Disability Research*. Leeds: The Disability Press.

Bond GR, Salyers MP, Rollins AL, Rapp CA & Zipple AM (2004) How evidence-based practices contribute to community integration. *Community Mental Health Journal* **4** (6) 569–588.

Brewis R (2007) *A Choice and a Voice*. Available at: http://www.in-control.org.uk (accessed June 2010).

Crane-Ross D, Roth D & Lauber BG (2000) Consumers' and case managers' perceptions of mental health and community support service needs. *Community Mental Health Journal* **36** (2) 161–178.

Department of Health (1999) *National Service Framework for Mental Health*. London: TSO.

Department of Health (2003) *Direct Payments Guidance: Community care, services for carers and children's services*. London: Department of Health.

Department of Health (2007) *Independence, Choice and Risk: A guide to best practice in supported decision making*. London: TSO.

Department of Health (2008) *Refocusing the Care Programme Approach: Policy and practice guidance*. London: TSO.

Department of Health (2009) *New Horizons: A shared vision for mental health*. London: TSO.

Frese FJ, Stanley J, Kress K & Vogel-Sciblia S (2001) Integrating evidence-based practices and the recovery model. *Psychiatric Services* **52** (11) 1462–1468.

Glendinning C, Challis D, Fernández JL, Jacobs S, Jones K, Knapp M, Manthorpe J, Moran N, Netten A, Stevens M & Wilberforce M (2008) *Evaluation of the Individual Budgets Pilot Programme: Summary report* [online]. SPRU/PSSRI/SCWRU. Available at: http://www.lse.ac.uk/collections/PSSRU/pdf/IBSENSummaryReport.pdf (accessed June 2010).

Kelly M & Gamble C (2005) Exploring the Concept of Recovery in Schizophrenia. *Journal of Psychiatric and Mental Health Nursing* **12** (2) 245–251.

MacKeith J & Burns S (2008) *Mental Health Recovery Star: User guide* [online]. Mental Health Providers Forum. Available at: http://www.mhpf.org.uk/recoveryStarResources.asp (accessed June 2010).

Manthorpe J, Stevens M, Challis D, Netten A, Glendinning C, Knapp M, Wilberforce M, Jacobs S, Jones K, Moran N & Fernandez J (2008) Individual budget projects come under the microscope. *Mental Health Today* Dec 22–26.

MIND (2009) *Personalisation in Mental Health: A review of the evidence* [online]. London: MIND. Available at: http://www.mind.org.uk/assets/0000/2164/putting_us_first_personalisation.pdf (accessed June 2010).

Morgan S (2000) *Clinical Risk Management: A clinical tool and practitioner manual*. London: SCMH.

National Institute for Clinical Excellence (NICE) (2010) *The NICE Guidelines on Core Interventions in the Treatment and Management of Schizophrenia in Adults in Primary and Secondary Care*. National Clinical Guideline No. 82. London: BPS/RCP.

Needham C & Carr S (2009) *Co-production: An emerging evidence base for adult social care transformation*. Research Briefing 31 [online]. London: SCIE. Available at: http://www.scie.org.uk/publications/briefings/files/briefing31.pdf (accessed June 2010).

Pawson R, Boaz A, Grayson L, Long A & Barnes C (2003) SCIE Knowledge review 03: *Types and quality of knowledge in Social Care* [online]. London: SCIE. Available at: http://www.scie.org.uk/publications/knowledgereviews/kr03.asp

RCP/SCIE (2007) *A Common Purpose: Recovery in future mental health services*. London: SCIE.

SCIE (2009) *At a Glance 18: Personalisation Briefing: Implications for community mental health services*. London: SCIE. Available at: http://www.scie.org.uk/publications/ataglance/ataglance18.pdf (accessed June 2010).

Spandler H & Vick N (2006) Opportunities for independent living using direct payments in mental health. *Health and Social Care in the Community* **14** (2) 107–115.

Stainton T & Boyce S (2004) I have got my life back: users' experience of direct payments. *Disability and Society* **19** (5) 443–454.

Tew J, Gould N, Abankwa D, Barnes H, Beresford P, Carr S, Copperman J, Ramon S, Rose D, Sweeney A & Woodward L (2006) *Values and Methodologies for Social Research in Mental Health*. London: SPN/NIMHE/SCIE. Available at: http://www.spn.org.uk/fileadmin/SPN_uploads/Documents/Values_and_methodologies.pdf (accessed June 2010).

Section 9: Promoting safety and positive risk taking

Empowering the person to decide the level of risk they are prepared to take with their health and safety. This includes working with the tension between promoting safety and positive risk taking, including assessing and dealing with possible risks for service users, carers, family members, and the wider public.

Risk assessment and risk management are currently central components of mental health services. Balancing the safety of the individual and wider society with the extension of choice and control and respect for self-determination is one of the skills that all mental health workers need to develop. However, the risk-averse culture that can dominate services has a tendency towards 'protection' at the expense of extending choice and enabling recovery, even where people have mental capacity to make choices of their own.

> *'Positive risk management as part of a carefully constructed plan is a desirable competence for all mental health practitioners, and will make risk management more effective. Over-defensive practice is bad practice. Avoiding all possible risks is not good for the service user or society in the long term ... creating more problems than it solves.'* (DH, 2007b, p8)

Positive risk taking has been an area of debate within mental health support for a number of years, with the link between an individual's right to take risks and their recovery outcomes being well evidenced (Ray *et al*, 2008; Morgan, 2004; RCP, 2008).

Aims

A personalised approach takes into account safety and safeguarding issues but places the control with the person and encourages a culture of positive risk and risk management that is based on partnership between the service user and the worker or service. As such, the overall aims of this section are:

- to explore the balance between safety and positive risk within the personalisation approach
- to consider how risk is perceived by different people/groups
- to create a direct link between recovery, positive risk and personalisation.

Overview

Safety and risk have been a focus of mental health services for many years, and the assessment and management of risk is an area of debate. The concept of positive risk has been identified as an area of good practice but is not fully implemented in services due to safety concerns and anxiety by professionals concerning the possible consequences.

Eleven areas of competence are included within this shared capability, these are:

Competence 1:	Demonstrate the ability to develop harmonious working relationships with service users and carers particularly with people who may not wish to engage with mental health services.
Competence 2:	Demonstrate and promote understanding of the factors associated with risk of harm to self or others through violence, self-neglect, self-harm or suicide.
Competence 3:	Demonstrate the ability to educate users and carers about the role, function and limitations of mental health services in relation to promoting safety and managing risk of harm.
Competence 4:	Contribute to accurate and effective risk assessments, identifying specific risk factors of relevance to the individual, their family and carers and the wider community (including risk of self-harm, self-neglect and violence to self or others).
Competence 5:	Contribute to the development of risk management strategies and plans, which involve the service user and name all the relevant people involved in their care and treatment and clearly identify the agreed actions to be taken and the goals to be achieved.
Competence 6:	Contribute, as a member of the therapeutic team, to the safe and effective management and reduction of any identified risks.
Competence 7:	Demonstrate knowledge and understanding of national and local policies and procedures for minimising risk and managing harm to self and others.
Competence 8:	Demonstrate knowledge and understanding of the care programme approach and its role in ensuring safe and effective care and treatment for service users and carers, particularly those who have a history of risks to self or others.
Competence 9:	Demonstrate understanding of the importance of multi-agency, multidisciplinary working in promoting safety and positive risk taking.
Competence 10:	Demonstrate awareness of the available spectrum of individual and service responses to help manage crises and minimise risks as they are happening eg. diffusion strategies, crisis response services.
Competence 11:	Contributing to use of medical and psychosocial interventions with the expressed goal of managing a person's risk behaviours in the long term eg. through use of medication, anger management, supportive counselling etc.

There has been a great deal of guidance and research into the area of risk in mental health, which it is useful for readers to be aware of. It must be noted that risk assessment is not an exact science, and while risk assessment and risk management plans should be linked, this does not fully mitigate against the risk.

From a personalisation perspective it is important that the service user is involved in any planning that occurs, and the process of risk assessment and management is a partnership between the person and their supporters, whether these are formal services or informal support arrangements. Introducing positive risk opportunities in a safe way needs full involvement and the traditional tick-box approach is not enough if choice and control is to be achieved.

This section of the workbook will assist readers to consider risk and safety and balance these with the aims of choice, control and positive risk within a personalised plan of support.

Competence 1

Demonstrate the ability to develop harmonious working relationships with service users and carers particularly with people who may wish not to engage with mental health services.

The ability to build relationships and rapport is a key skill for all those involved in mental health service delivery, and is an area that has been shown to contribute to the individual's recovery (Howgego *et al*, 2003; McCabe & Priebe, 2004; Hewitt & Coffey, 2005). Within a personalised approach this relationship should be dictated by the service user. However, within the mental health context this is not always the case, and assertive approaches to engagement have been developed which at times provide little choice for the person in terms of whether they have contact with the service or not. The dilemma of this situation is not something that is debated here, however, the forming of relationships and the issue of engagement is a competence that needs to be a central skill for all those providing services.

Engagement is a term that is often used in mental health settings and it can be used in a detrimental context. It seems that services often blame the individual rather than asking why and how the service can engage with the person. Personalisation should turn this situation on its head, with engagement being the joint responsibility of the person and the support mechanisms, rather than it being solely the responsibility of the person. Issues such as times of operation, the service being offered and the relationship with the key worker are all areas that need to be considered if the service is to be tailored to individual needs and preferences.

The reasons that individuals do not engage with services or the reasons why services do not engage with the person are varied. A review undertaken by the Sainsbury Centre for Mental Health (SCMH) in 1998 identified some of these reasons included:

> *'...individual experiences ... inappropriate nature of services ... suspicious of statutory services ... services have little to offer or may have experienced negative staff attitudes. Services may find it difficult to engage because they are too focused on immediate outcomes or on medical treatment alone, or because they lack the staff with the appropriate skills and the time or resources to achieve engagement.'* (SCMH, 1998, p8)

While this review is now quite old, the reasons why people do not take up services remain valid and need to be considered in the engagement process.

Reflection points

- How do you approach making a relationship with a person you are working with?
- How does this approach encourage engagement?

Assertive outreach approaches were made a requirement of mental health services by the National Service Framework (DH, 1999) and the subsequent NHS Plan (DH, 2000), which set out the need for services to take an assertive and more flexible approach to treatment for those who have multiple and complex needs and who have traditionally not taken up the services offered by mainstream mental health provision. Key elements of the approach are being introduced across other services, including seeing service users in a range of settings according to where they feel most comfortable, and as personalisation progresses, this creativity and flexibility will need to further increase, as per the demands of those who access this type of support.

From a personalisation perspective, this is a tension within the delivery of support, and while user choice and control are central principles of the approach there will be instances where the choice to access a service is not as negotiable as it may be with other service user groups. This tension needs careful consideration if the relationship is to be developed and engagement from both the service user and the worker is to be promoted.

Case study exercise

Stuart is a gay man in his mid-30s. He has a long-term partner who he lives with and he works part-time at the local night shelter. He has experienced mental health difficulties for a number of years and does not like seeing anyone from the mental health team. He says that the service makes him feel helpless and out of control, and he says the team do not involve his partner which he finds offensive. Following a family bereavement, Stuart is finding it difficult to cope; he is not sleeping, not eating very well, and is very anxious.

Stuart recognises that he needs some support but is suspicious of the team; he says he does not want to take any medication and doesn't like to be seen at the team's offices as he feels people will know what he is there for.

- What approach would you take to encourage Stuart to engage with the service?

One approach that has been developed as part of personalisation is that of risk enablement, which forms part of the support planning process. Risk enablement refers to a part of the support planning process that includes the person and their supporters considering the assessment, understanding and possible management of risks (Tyson *et al*, 2010). This takes a person-centred view of the issues and encourages shared ownership of the risks and any mitigating plans, as well as ensuring that any plans are appropriate to the situation.

'A person-centred approach to risk uses questions around a framework of purpose, people, process and progress – it is important that right at the beginning of the process we think seriously about what it is we are trying to achieve. Our thinking about how the process can be used to enable the person to have choice and control in their life, and to be a citizen in the community, will influence who the people are that are called to participate in the process.' (Neill *et al*, 2008, p11)

Risk enablement panels have been established in some areas to support the process. These are forums that often sit with local authority safeguarding teams, and which can convene if there are complex risks that need to be considered before agreeing a support plan. The aim is to create an environment where the risks can be fully discussed and any management plans identified and agreed, and they involve the individual, their supporters, service providers and any other relevant individuals.

Competence 2

Demonstrate and promote understanding of the factors associated with risk of harm to self or others through violence, self-neglect, self-harm or suicide.

Risk of harm is the main focus in the majority of risk assessment processes and most risk assessments will consist of a number of factors which impact on the risk of violence, neglect, self-harm and suicide, and being aware of these is useful knowledge. However, it should be noted that identifying these factors and implementing management plans do not guarantee that harm will not occur and this view of clinical risk can be limiting, with the wider social situations and the individual's rights to self-determination being ignored or minimised as a result of the approach.

In terms of violence to others, there is significant research that suggests that those with mental health problems are no more prone to violence than the general population (Stuart, 2003; Wessely, 1993). However, there is research that suggests that violence is more common among those with mental health issues (Wessely, 1993; Choe *et al*, 2008). Self-neglect is a far more common occurrence than violence and it is estimated that 0.5 per 1,000 of the population (Day & Leahy-Warren, 2008) experiences self-neglect. Self-harm and suicide is often dealt with together; however, these are often separate issues. Self-harming behaviour tends to be as a result of emotional distress, with actions such as cutting, burning or poisoning, which is not intended to be life threatening and is often repeated (Rethink, 2007). Whereas suicidal thoughts or behaviour tend to be more as a result of a sense of hopelessness and is usually a deliberate and planned act (MIND, 2008).

Regardless of whether the incidences are higher or not there remains a lot of stigma around mental health problems and harm (SHIFT, 2008; Blumenthal & Lavender, 2001; DH, 2009), which has a significant impact on both individuals and the way services respond. The impact of social exclusion and stigma was discussed in detail in section 4, however, it is also important here, as the traditional views of risk and harm can create real obstacles in the implementation of a personalised approach.

Research into self-directed support has highlighted that there is a lower likelihood of people being offered direct payments and personal budgets as a result of professional assumptions and anxieties concerning risk and perceptions about the person's capacity. The evaluation of the individual budgets pilots (Glendinning *et al*, 2008) found that while there was no apparent increased risk to or by people using individual budgets, worker concerns about the risk of neglect, financial abuse and physical harm did increase. The assumptions around personalised options in mental health appear to be based on anxiety about negative consequences. However, the evidence shows that people with mental health issues using individual budgets experience an increase in both quality of life and overall well-being (NMHDU, 2010; Duffy, 2010). Balancing the 'duty of care' and the ability of services to safeguard individuals is often carried out at the cost of promoting choice, control and independence. There needs to be a shift towards enabling the person to take the risks that would allow them to lead a more active, self-determined and independent life and to identify and report any concerns they have about keeping safe as a part of the overall support planning. This is a different way of working than has previously been the case, however, it is also one which has many benefits in terms of managing the wide variety of risks and emphasising self-determination of the individual and supporting the individual's recovery.

Reflection point

How do you decide which risks are acceptable and which are not?

The traditional view of risk is often limited, considering only the clinical view of harm to self or others, whereas in mental health terms there is a much wider debate to be had if positive risk is to become a real opportunity. Risk in a personalised mental health setting is not solely about harm, it should also take account of the opportunities for positive risk taking, the use of individual resources to manage issues as they arise, the risk of intervening and the views and perspectives of the individual and their supporters.

The framework for self-directed support, which includes discussion and review of the individual's concerns and aspirations about risk and an understanding of their social and environmental context as well as their coping strategies, is one of the means of promoting positive risk and self-determination of individuals. For people with mental health problems, this should also include supportive discussion about things like self-harm or substance use. Control rather than prevention, is an approach that has been supported by many service users, and these types of strategies, with mechanisms for reporting and exploring concerns, need to be built into support plans. This is also supported by the government guidance *Independence, Choice and Risk* (DH, 2007a), which recommends the following approach to risk management:

> '*...that people have the right to live their lives to the full as long as that does not stop others from doing the same.* (DH, 2007a, p3)

Competence 3

Demonstrate the ability to educate users and carers about the role, function and limitations of mental health services in relation to promoting safety and managing risk of harm.

Information is an important element in personalisation, and individuals need to understand what is available and the roles that different services may play in order to make an informed choice about what support options they access. The brokerage role within a personalised model will help to ensure current information is available, however, this is being approached differently across the country and in some areas is not independent from local authorities or not fully implemented. Brokerage is a term that is used to mean the individual or service that helps to identify and purchase support packages, sometimes this includes advocacy and ongoing support and sometimes it is solely a source of information and advice. In each area individuals will need to familiarise themselves with what type of brokerage is available as this is key to ensuring choice and control in the support planning process.

The role of the NHS and local authority services is set to change as personalisation is implemented, and this is an area that has been extensively debated (Williams, 2009; Needham, 2009; Scourfield, 2008). Local interpretation will define the services role. However, the emphasis is towards facilitating and supporting individuals to access more universal and community services. In terms of risk assessment and management, the initial risk assessment and management processes may well still be undertaken by local authority and NHS staff, as these are the services that provide access to funding for support packages. The NHS and Community Care Act (1990) places a duty on social services departments to carry out an assessment of need for eligibility for social care support, and this legislation is not set to change at this time. As such, individuals will still need to have contact with statutory services to be able to access direct payments or individual budgets.

Assessment and management of risk does not mean that the risk can be removed, and while services can identify issues and help people to manage difficult situations they cannot guarantee safety in all cases or protect people from all harm. Risk is a factor in everybody's lives and this is no different when the person has mental health problems. The sharing of risk assessment and management between individual and service can help to manage the situation better by introducing personal ownership into the process and enabling the person to take more control of their situation.

Reflection point

How do you ensure that the person is aware of the roles and functions of the service?

The Mental Capacity Act (2005) (MCA) provides a useful framework for thinking about risk taking and decision making that is based on five principles, these are:

- a presumption of capacity
- individuals being supported to make their own decisions
- people have the right to make unwise decisions
- any decisions taken on behalf of someone without capacity is in their best interests
- any decision applies the least restrictive option in the circumstances.

Presumptions about capacity are identified as a barrier to the uptake of direct payments in mental health, and as such the MCA can be a useful tool to consider whether the individual first, has capacity, and second is being supported to make decisions for themselves. This applies to issues about risk that may be evident, and supports the principle that individuals have the right to make decisions and must be supported to consider the risks and the impact of their choices.

Reflection point

How can the principles of the MCA help you to consider decisions about risk?

One further element of risk that is often not fully considered but which can have significant impact upon an individual's well-being and their overall recovery, is the risk that the services themselves present. Work carried out in the *Pathways to Personalisation* project (NMHDU, 2010) included interviews with service users concerning their views of risk, and a range of issues were identified that were as a direct result of using mental health services. These included discrimination as a result of using mental health services and personal safety while staying on inpatient units, among others, and created real concerns and barriers for individuals. When considering personalised approaches this is an important area that needs to be considered and balanced with any action that is taken. Different means of support, such as direct payments and personal budgets, can be used to support an individual who may be experiencing crisis in a way that is more appropriate to their wishes and preferences.

Competence 4

Contribute to accurate and effective risk assessments, identifying specific risk factors of relevance to the individual, their family and carers and the wider community (including risk of self-harm, self-neglect and violence to self or others).

The definition of risk is that an outcome is uncertain, however, this is largely viewed as a negative outcome within mental health services and the aim is generally to protect against these negative outcomes. This is not always possible or desirable (DH, 2007b), and positive risk also needs to be considered with the person as part of the support planning process. In addition, how a person perceives whether something is a risk or not depends on a wide variety of factors and the social and psychological context of a person will influence how a risk is seen and whether that risk is taken. Social factors, cultural beliefs, and lifestyle choices can all impact upon what is seen as risky and these need to be identified within the process to ensure that individuals and supporters have a shared understanding of what risk means in that person's context.

There is a whole range of risk assessment tools available, and what is used in each area is different, however, there are a number of common themes. These themes largely relate to the risk of harm to self and others, and the person's vulnerability to abuse or exploitation. This approach can be a barrier in itself, and focuses on the negative aspects of clinical risk rather than the individual and their supporters' views and strengths. The views of carers are often very different from those of the individual themself and this is something that needs to be managed as part of the process. By applying the framework of self-directed support and encouraging open conversation with both the individual and their support network it is possible to consider all the varying views and agree on a support plan that enables positive risk and provides a safety net for the individual.

Case study exercise

Jane is a 23-year old single woman. She is from an orthodox Jewish background but is not particularly religious now and has not been to synagogue for several years. Jane has had several short-term relationships and her last partner was violent towards her, which resulted in her being assaulted and admitted to hospital for a week with fractures and bruising. Jane does not have contact with her family and has very few friends who she sees regularly. She is unemployed and claims incapacity benefit and disability living allowance, she has no formal qualifications and does not know what she wants to do.

Jane has been in contact with the mental health team for several years and has a diagnosis of borderline personality disorder, she regularly self-harms by cutting herself, and uses drugs and alcohol often. She also often goes out to pubs and clubs to pick up men for casual sex.

Jane is currently quite low in mood and says she is struggling to sleep or generally take care of herself. She says she is bored and lonely and *'just doesn't see the point in anything'* at the moment.

- What are the possible risks that need to be included within Jane's support plan?

- How would you support her to manage these issues?

Competence 5

Contribute to the development of risk management strategies and plans, which involve the service user and name all the relevant people involved in their care and treatment and clearly identify the agreed actions to be taken and the goals to be achieved.

The involvement of service users and their friends and family in risk assessment and management is a key element of the support planning processes within a personalised approach, and the guidance states that the risk management plan should be a shared tool (DH, 2007a; 2007b) and not simply a professional exercise. In the context of promoting independence, the individual has the right to take risks, and within the MCA framework, which presumes capacity, also has the right to make decisions that may be considered unwise. The role of the support planning process is to provide an opportunity to identify, discuss and plan any safeguards that might help to support the individual. This is not a process of professional leadership but rather one where the service user is central and in control.

Partnership in this process is something which cannot only increase the person's control and sense of responsibility, but also may help to combat the risk-averse nature of services as new ways of managing risks can be identified and the ownership shared (Tait & Lester, 2005; Ray *et al*, 2008; Morgan, 2000).

> *'Risk management should be conducted in a spirit of collaboration and based on a relationship between the service user and their carers that is as trusting as possible.'* (DH, 2007b, p5)

In current practice environments there appears to be an emphasis on the negatives of risk, and by exploring these with the person(s) concerned, opportunities for positive risk can be identified. Protective factors, such as the person's strengths and resources, can be highlighted to introduce self-management into their care and support plan and encourage personal control into the process.

Service user involvement in mental health care has traditionally been patchy (Langan & Lindow, 2004; Tait & Lester, 2005), and personalisation should help to change this by placing a requirement on service providers to deliver a system that offers choice and control to the person accessing services.

Reflection point

How do you make sure the individual has choice and control in the risk assessment and management processes?

Risk management plans need to be a working document, which can be adapted as the person's situation changes. They should be based upon the individual's goals and provide strategies to safeguard the person where this is needed and agreed. Involving the person and their support system is an important factor in this process as they are the ones who have knowledge and experience of the situation and the types of triggers and coping strategies that have previously been effective. The self-directed support framework, which includes regular reviews, provides an opportunity for this to be achieved, and risk should be embedded within the overall support plan.

Competence 6

Contribute, as a member of the therapeutic team, to the safe and effective management and reduction of any identified risks.

Multidisciplinary working has been best practice guidance in mental health for many years, and in addition to involvement and shared ownership of risk with the individual it is also recommended that risk assessment and management is shared across the team involved in the person's support. Within a personalised plan this may involve a range of roles, services, and informal supporters, and workers will need to ensure they include all those involved and there is a clarity about who is providing support to manage any risks.

Contingency and crisis planning is a part of the Care Programme Approach (CPA) (DH, 2008), and a way in which individuals can exercise choice and control in situations which may be largely out of their immediate control. Agreeing a plan of action, should the risk become too high to manage, including what threshold is being used to determine this, and how the person would like their situation to be handled if there is a crisis, is an important factor in both recovery and personalisation as it retains the person as central to the support plan and uses their goals, preferences and wishes as the foundation for any crisis interventions.

The identification of risks both positive and negative should be a central part of the planning that takes place, and risks of relapse in mental health and any risks to the person achieving their goals should also be part of the assessment process. Regardless of the role an individual may be playing within the person's life, they will have a role in the management and reduction of risk. Sharing information and creating a relationship, in which the person can talk about and explore their strengths and needs, are a key part of effective risk management.

Case study exercise

James is a 35-year-old man from an African-Caribbean background. He was born in England shortly after his parents immigrated. James is diagnosed with schizophrenia and has had several hospital admissions due to episodes of psychosis when he becomes very paranoid and agitated.

James currently lives in a self-contained flat in the town centre. He likes his flat and has spent time decorating it but says that the area is not very good and is very worried about being broken into or his place getting vandalised.

James has a large family, his parents live locally and he has five brothers, a sister and his grandmother lives with his parents. He has contact with all of his family and says he is particularly close to his mother and youngest brother.

James has worked in the past, most recently as a painter and decorator, a job he would like to go back to. He is currently doing a work experience placement with a local employer and is hoping that this will develop into something more permanent but he is concerned that his mental health diagnosis might go against him and is anxious about this.

James has a care co-ordinator from the local community mental health team and has a direct payment, which he uses for transport to get him to his work placement. He also sees a support worker once a week who has been helping him to access local sports activities and a housing support worker who helps him with his flat and the associated bills.

- Who needs to be involved in James's plan?

- How would you make sure James is able to control and manage his own risks?

Competence 7

Demonstrate knowledge and understanding of national and local policies and procedures for minimising risk and managing harm to self and others.

Each local area or service will have its own policies and procedures on risk assessment and management, and those involved with the delivery of these should make themselves aware of the framework in which they are operating as a basic competence requirement. In terms of national policy and procedure, there have been a number of guidance documents published to guide practice in this area.

The 2007 Department of Health publication *Best Practice in Managing Risk* is the significant policy development and this document is referred to across mental health policy. Other guidance and research is available when considering capacity and particular issues (DH, 2007a; Ray *et al*, 2008; DH, 2008). However, the best practice guidance is the framework in which mental health services largely operate.

Best practice in managing risk identifies a number of practice points that need to be in place, these are largely consistent with the personalised approach and those involved in the process with an individual should apply the following principles.

- Decisions should be based on knowledge of the individual service user and their social context, knowledge of the service user's own experience, and professional judgement.

- Positive risk management as part of a carefully constructed plan is a required competence for all mental health practitioners.
- Risk management should be conducted in a spirit of collaboration and based on a relationship between the service user and their carers that is as trusting as possible.
- Risk management must be built on recognition of the service user's strengths and should emphasise recovery.
- Risk management involves developing flexible strategies aimed at preventing any negative event from occurring or, if this is not possible, minimising the harm caused.
- Risk management should take into account that risk can be both general and specific, and that good management can reduce and prevent harm.
- The risk management plan should include a summary of all risks identified, formulations of the situations in which identified risks may occur, and actions to be taken by practitioners and the service user in response to crisis.
- All staff involved in risk management must be capable of demonstrating sensitivity and competence in relation to diversity in race, faith, age, gender, disability and sexual orientation.
- Risk management must always be based on awareness of the capacity for the service user's risk level to change over time, and recognition that each service user requires a consistent and individualised approach.
- A risk management plan is only as good as the time and effort put into communicating its findings to others. (Adapted from: DH, 2007b, p5–6)

These points cover both involvement and positive risk and provide a good basis on which to develop a personalised risk assessment and management plan as they recognise that each individual's situation is different and an individual approach is needed.

Case study exercise

Dermot is from southern Ireland and moved to England five years ago. He is from a strict Catholic family. He has recently turned 30 and is starting to get concerned about what he is going to do with his life. He has had a series of short-term jobs and is currently working as a barman in a local pub. He has a history of heavy drinking but is not drinking at the moment and says he wants to keep it that way.

Dermot has previously been in contact with mental health services. When he first came out to his family as being gay and moved to England, he went through a period of depression and harmed himself by burning his thighs with cigarettes. He says he still does this on occasion but never bad enough to need treatment and it helps him to feel calmer.

He is not in contact with his family since he came out to them as it was not received well. His father, in particular, was very angry and Dermot feels that he has been rejected. He would like to make contact with his mother and sister but says that he is scared of his father's reaction to him. His mother has written to him once a month since he moved. Dermot has a group of close friends and he works with two of them at his bar job. He says that there is one man at his work who he finds attractive and would like to explore a possible relationship.

- What are the risks in Dermot's case?
- What are the strengths or protective factors that Dermot has to draw upon?
- Draw up an initial risk management plan based on these – identifying the opportunities for positive risk in this case.

The framework provided by the 2007 document *Independence Choice and Risk* (DH, 2007a), which should be considered alongside the best practice guidance and also the principles of the MCA, is a further useful tool when considering risk. This guidance considered how individuals are best supported to make decisions about risks for themselves, while providing a safety net that safeguards when needed, and several principles were identified to guide this process, these are:

- help people to have choice and control over their lives
- recognise that making a choice can sometimes involve an element of risk
- help people to understand their responsibilities and the implications of their choices, including any risks
- acknowledge that there will often be some risk, and that trying to remove it altogether can outweigh the quality of life benefits for the person. (DH, 2007b, p9)

Reflection point

How can these frameworks support decisions about risk and create a more personalised approach to risk management?

Competence 8

Demonstrate knowledge and understanding of the care programme approach and its role in ensuring safe and effective care and treatment for service users and carers, particularly those who have a history of risks to self or others.

The Care Programme Approach (CPA) was initially introduced into mental health services in 1991 as a case management approach for people with severe mental health difficulties. Its aim was to provide a comprehensive and co-ordinated approach to support, however, this was not universally achieved and while it did improve the contact services had with people in the community, it was not the revolution in service delivery that was intended (Simpson *et al*, 2003a; Simpson *et al*, 2003b; Kingdon & Amanullah, 2005). In 2006 the Department of Health launched a consultation on reforming the CPA system and in 2008 *Refocusing the Care Programme Approach*, was published. The 2008 guidance is the current position, and highlights what should be in place to deliver a CPA approach within mental health services. One of the positive developments with the 2008 CPA guidance is that is sets out the principles and values that should guide case management in mental health, and these consider personalisation, social inclusion and individual rights as central elements of the approach.

Principles of CPA

- The individual is central to the support process.
- Social inclusion and recovery are promoted.
- Strengths, goals and aspirations should be explored and included, as well as needs and difficulties.
- It recognises the individual as a person first and patient/service user second.
- Assessment and planning views a person 'in the round' seeing and supporting them in their individual diverse roles and the multiple needs they have, with the aim of promoting well-being.
- Self-care is promoted and supported wherever possible.
- Action is taken to encourage independence and self-determination.
- Carers form a vital part of the support required to aid a person's recovery. Their own needs should also be recognised and supported.
- Services should be organised and delivered in ways that promote and co-ordinate helpful and purposeful mental health practice based on fulfilling therapeutic relationships and partnerships between the people involved.

(Adapted from: DH, 2008, p7)

CPA as an approach is designed to consider strengths, goals, complexity of needs and risks, and as a case management tool can contribute to the delivery of safe and effective care. However, this is dependent upon communication and implementation of the approach, which can be variable.

The principles of CPA are to provide a co-ordinated approach, to join-up the various individuals and services involved in supporting a person and to make sure that the care and support a person accesses is appropriate for their needs. For those with multiple services involved or particularly complex needs CPA provides a framework in which the whole person is considered and a plan is drawn up. The involvement of individuals and their support networks is part of this framework, and other services such as those purchased with direct payments or individual budgets, or community supports should also be involved, and named, in the support or risk management plans as appropriate and agreed with the person.

Reflection point

How do you make sure that communication is maintained and support is joined-up when there are several people or services involved in providing support?

The support planning processes within the framework of self-directed support is complementary to CPA and develops the process further by ensuring that the individual and their carers/supporters become central to the review processes. Within this framework it is possible to provide both opportunity and safeguards as the co-productive relationship supports communication and problem solving.

Competence 9

Demonstrate understanding of the importance of multi-agency, multidisciplinary working in promoting safety and positive risk taking.

In a care and support plan, where a number of services or professionals are involved, communication becomes an essential skill for all parties. The input of different stakeholders can improve both safeguarding and the ability to introduce positive risk into a plan as it provides a wider network on which to draw, and a range of support possibilities. While team working allows for sharing knowledge about the individual and their situation from different perspectives, including the person's own, there is also the potential for conflicting views about risk and these needs to be openly discussed and explored. In a service which is risk-averse it can be a challenge to introduce the idea of positive risk and the rights of individuals to take risks, however, for personalisation to succeed this must be challenged.

Positive risk does not mean that risks are ignored or avoided, but rather that the consequences are carefully weighed up and a plan is developed to support the desired goal and minimise harmful outcomes (Morgan, 2004). Responsibility and shared ownership is a vital part of this process as the individual needs to be fully engaged with shaping the plan.

'Getting the balance right between creativity, personal control, aspiration and positive risk management is a key challenge to address for personalisation. Risk is something we all live with every day and is an important part of opportunity and change but responses to this in services can sometimes result in over-restrictive practices.' (NMHDU, 2010, p11)

An individual's strengths and needs are identified and previous experiences of what works can be drawn on to inform the actions, with the emphasis being on informed choice and maximising opportunities for independence. The process of positive risk involves being open and honest about risks and considering the range of views, which may at times conflict with each other. The frameworks of *Independence, Choice and Risk* (DH, 2007a) and the MCA both indicate that individuals have the right to take risks and these should be supported with the emphasis being on providing a safety net and ensuring that choices are based on informed decisions, in which the individual is supported to consider all of the possible consequences and benefits of their actions.

Reflection points

- How do you support a person in making an informed choice?
- Consider an example of positive risk in your experience. How was this planned and how were the concerns about safety addressed?

Competence 10

Demonstrate awareness of the available spectrum of individual and service responses to help manage crises and minimise risks as they are happening eg. diffusion strategies, crisis response services.

Crisis services were introduced consistently across NHS and social care services at the same time as assertive outreach services by the NSF (DH, 1999) and NHS plan (DH, 2000). These services were intended to be multidisciplinary and to provide intensive support at times when people were struggling in order to avoid hospital admission. This model is one which has been used with some success, and which can respond in a much more flexible and creative way than community teams. Third sector providers, such as MIND, have provided crisis housing and other support services for some time and it may be that in many cases the crisis event is as a result of social difficulties, which need this type of response, rather than an acute mental health problem.

Reflection point

What services are available in your area to help to manage crisis and risk?

Applying a personalised approach at times of crisis is a shift in the way services have traditionally responded, and this is something that needs to be considered. Crisis services and intensive support have been shown to help people at times of distress (Roberts, 2005; Flannery & Everly, 2000). However, within a personalised approach these need to be delivered in a way which meets the preferences of the individual. Crisis and contingency planning is one way in which a person can retain some control in times of crisis and advanced statements and directives are also an option that can be used to enable the person to set out what they want to happen if a crisis occurs.

An advanced directive is a decision that has legal status and can only be used to refuse a specific treatment in a specific situation, an advanced statement on the other hand can be used as part of the CPA documents and sets out the preferences and wishes of the person at times of crisis or when they may be unable to make the decision for themselves. These two tools should not be confused, as legally, an advanced directive is usually binding, whereas an advanced statement is effectively a crisis and contingency plan and can specify a whole range of wishes and preferences, which should be considered.

Reflection point

If you were drawing up an advanced statement or contingency plan for yourself what would you include?

Competence 11

Contributing to use of medical and psychosocial interventions with the expressed goal of managing a person's risk behaviours in the long term eg. through use of medication, anger management, supportive counselling etc.

There is a range of treatments and support available for mental health issues, and personalisation will increase the choices around how and what is accessed and provided. From a recovery perspective medical, psychological and social issues are all considered and as such, workers need to have an overview of the various options and be able to provide the relevant information to enable individuals to make an informed choice about their support options. The term psychosocial interventions is used to mean a range of treatments that take a psychological and social focus to help people to cope with and manage difficulties including symptoms of mental health problems, structuring the day, changing behaviours and managing relationship and communication difficulties.

The most common forms of psychosocial treatments that are used within mental health services are psycho-education, family work and cognitive behaviour therapy, although other interventions such as coping skills, stress management and motivational work are also commonly available. Talking therapies have been a focus of mental health services for some time, with psychosocial interventions being recommended for use with psychosis and other mental health difficulties (Pinquart & Sorenson, 2001; Brooker, 2001; Harris *et al*, 2002; Cleary *et al*, 2008). These interventions can help people cope with a wide range of issues and each person's plan needs to be tailored to their particular needs to determine what might work. There is an evidence base for these approaches, however, this needs to be approached with caution, as discussed in section 8, to ensure that individual preferences are considered and a personalised approach is taken. Using psychosocial interventions to manage risk has been shown to be effective (Brooker, 2001; Turkington *et al*, 2006; Pilling *et al*, 2002) with behaviour change being the main focus. Improved family relationships, increased agreement with treatment plans and improved self-management are just some of the outcomes that have been demonstrated, and these interventions are also considered to be cost-effective – with a range of workers receiving additional training and supervision to be able to deliver talking therapies in a range of settings.

Reflection points

- What interventions are available in your area or service?
- How do you ensure that individuals are able to make an informed choice about what intervention or treatment they want and need?

Summary

This capability has considered several issues relating to risk and safety in mental health support and how this is balanced with the individual's rights and a personalised approach, which emphasises service user choice and control. The competency for this shared capability is:

'Empowering the person to decide the level of risk they are prepared to take with their health and safety. This includes working with the tension between promoting safety and positive risk taking, including assessing and dealing with possible risks for service users, carers, family members, and the wider public.'

Risk is a subjective concept, with social context, attitudes and beliefs all impacting upon whether something is seen as a risk or not. There is increasing focus on positive risk in mental health, which supports both the recovery and personalisation approaches, and places the individual as central to the support by recognising that risks can also be opportunities. This is a shift in the traditional risk-averse culture of mental health support and one that services are struggling to implement.

Personalisation is an approach that considers people's rights and responsibilities, and taking a partnership approach, which seeks to share the risk between the service user and the service in the assessment and management processes, is one way in which individuals can exercise increased choice and control to meet their needs and aspirations.

Summary exercise

Write a short summary of what this capability means to you in your context/practice, and then answer the following three questions.

- What have you learnt by completing this section?

- How have you now reached competence in this area?

- What do you need to do to maintain your competence?

References

Blumenthal S & Lavender T (2001) *Violence and Mental Disorder: A critical aid to the assessment and management of risk*. London: Jessica Kingsley/Zito Trust.

Brooker C (2001) A decade of evidence-based training for work with people with serious mental health problems: progress in the development of psychosocial interventions. *Journal of Mental Health* **10** (1) 17–31.

Choe JY, Teplin LA & Abram KM (2008) Perpetration of violence, violent victimization, and severe mental illness: balancing public health concerns. *Psychiatric Services* **59** 153–164.

Cleary M, Hunt GE, Matheson SL, Siegfried N & Walter G (2008) Psychosocial interventions for people with both severe mental illness and substance misuse. *Cochrane Database of Systematic Reviews 2008*, Issue 1. Art. No. CD001088. DOI: 10.1002/14651858.CD001088.pub2.

Day MR & Leahy-Warren P (2008) Self-neglect 1: recognising features & risk factors. *Nursing Times* **104** (24) 26–27.

Department of Health (1999) *National Service Framework for Mental Health: Modern standards and service models*. London: TSO.

Department of Health (2000) *The NHS Plan: A plan for investment, A plan for reform*. London: TSO.

Department of Health (2007a) *Independence, Choice and Risk: A guide to best practice in supported decision-making*. London: TSO.

Department of Health (2007b) *Best Practice in Managing Risk: Principles and guidance for best practice in the assessment and management of risk to self and others in mental health services*. London: TSO.

Department of Health (2008) *Refocusing the Care Programme Approach: Policy and practice guidance*. London: TSO.

Department of Health (2009) *Attitudes to Mental Illness research report 2009* [online]. London: DH. Available at: http://www.dh.gov.uk/en/Publicationsandstatistics/PublishedSurvey/ListOfSurveySince1990/Surveylistmentalhealth/index.htm (accessed June 2010).

Duffy S (2010) *Personalisation in Mental Health*. Sheffield: Centre for Welfare Reform/ Yorkshire & Humberside Improvement Partnership, Care Pathways & Packages Project & ADASS.

Flannery RB & Everly GS (2000) Crisis intervention: A review. *International Journal of Emergency Mental Health* **2** (2) 119–125.

Glendinning C, Challis D, Fernandez J-L, Jacobs S, Jones K, Knapp M, Manthorpe J, Moran N, Netten A, Stevens M & Wilberforce M (2008) *Evaluation of the Individual Budgets Pilot Programme: Final report*. London: SPRU/PSSRU/SCWRU.

Harris N, Williams S & Bradshaw T (Eds) (2002) *Psychosocial Interventions for People with Schizophrenia: A practical guide for mental health workers*. Basingstoke: Palgrave Macmillan.

Hewitt J & Coffey M (2005) Therapeutic working relationships with people with schizophrenia: literature review. *Journal of Advanced Nursing* **52** (5) 561–570.

Howgego IM, Yellowless P, Owen C, Meldrum L & Dark F (2003) The therapeutic alliance: the key to effective patient outcome? A descriptive review of the evidence in community mental health case management. *Australian and New Zealand Journal of Psychiatry* **37** (2) 169–183.

Kingdon D & Amanullah S (2005) Care programme approach: relapsing or recovering? *Advances in Psychiatric Treatment* **11** 325–329.

Langan J & Lindow V (2004) *Living with Risk: Mental health service user involvement in risk assessment and management*. Bristol: Policy Press.

McCabe R & Priebe S (2004) The Therapeutic Relationship in the Treatment of Severe Mental Illness: A review of methods and findings. *International Journal of Social Psychiatry* **50** (2) 115–128.

MIND (2008) *How to Help Someone Who is Suicidal* [online]. Available at: http://www.mind.org.uk/help/medical_and_alternative_care/how_to_help_someone_who_is_suicidal#selfharm (accessed June 2010).

Morgan S (2000) *Clinical Risk Management: A clinical tool and practitioner manual*. London: The Sainsbury Centre for Mental Health.

Morgan S (2004) Positive risk-taking: an idea whose time has come. *Health Care Risk Report* **October** 18–19.

Needham C (2009) Interpreting personalisation in England's National Health Service: a textual analysis. *Critical Policy Studies* **3** (2) 204–220.

Neill M, Allen J, Woodhead N, Reif S, Irwin L & Sanderson H (2008) *A Positive Approach to Risk Requires Person Centred Thinking* [online]. Available at: http://www.dhcarenetworks.org.uk/--_library/Resources/Personalisation/Personalisation_advice/A_Person_Centred_Approach_to_Risk.pdf (accessed June 2010).

NMHDU (2010) *Paths to Personalisation in Mental Health: A whole system, whole life framework* [online]. London: DH. Available at: http://www.nmhdu.org.uk/resources/personalisation-in-mental-health-emerging-programme/paths-to-personalisation (accessed June 2010).

Pilling S, Bebbington P, Kuipers E, Garety P, Geddes J, Orbach G & Morgan C (2002) Psychological treatments in schizophrenia: I. Meta-analysis of family intervention and cognitive behaviour therapy. *Psychological Medicine* **32** (5) 763–782.

Pinquart M & Sorenson S (2001) How effective are psychotherapeutic and other psychosocial interventions with older adults? *Journal of Mental Health and Aging* **7** (2) 207–243.

Ray M, Pugh R, Roberts D & Beech B (2008) *Mental Health and Social Work*. Research Briefing 26. London: SCIE.

Rethink (2007) *Suicide and Self Harm* [online]. Available at: http://www.rethink.org/living_with_mental_illness/coping_in_a_crisis/suicide_self_harm/index.html (accessed June 2010).

Roberts A (2005) *Crisis Intervention Handbook: Assessment, treatment and research*. Oxford: Oxford University Press.

Royal College of Psychiatrists (RCP) (2008) *Rethinking Risk to Others in Mental Health Services*. College report CR150. London: RCP.

SCMH (1998) *Keys to Engagement: Review of carers for people with severe mental illness who are hard to engage with service*. London: SCMH.

Scourfield P (2008) Going for brokerage: a task of 'independent support' or social work? *British Journal of Social Work* **40** (3) 858–877.

SHIFT (2008) *What's the Story? Reporting mental health and suicide*. London: SHIFT.

Simpson A, Miller C & Bowers L (2003a) The history of the Care Programme Approach in England: where did it go wrong? *Journal of Mental Health* **12** (6) 489–504.

Simpson A, Miller C & Bowers L (2003b) Case management models and the care programme approach: how to make the CPA effective and credible. *Journal of Psychiatric and Mental Health Nursing* **10** 472–483.

Stuart H (2003) Violence and mental illness: an overview. *World Psychiatry* **2** (2) 121–124.

Tait L & Lester H (2005) Encouraging user involvement in mental health services. *Advances in Psychiatric Treatment* **11** 168–175.

Tyson A, Brewis R, Crosby N, Hatton C, Stansfield J, Tomlinson C, Waters J & Wood A (2010) *In Control Third Phase: Evaluation and learning 2008–2009*. London: In Control.

Turkington D, Kingdon D, Rathod S, Hammond K., Pelton J & Mehta R (2006) Outcomes of an effectiveness trial of cognitive-behavioural intervention by mental health nurses in schizophrenia. *British Journal of Psychiatry* **186** 36–40.

Wessely S (1993) Violence and psychosis. In: C Thompson & P Cowen (Eds). *Violence. Basic and clinical science*. Oxford: Butterworth/Heinemann.

Williams C (2009) Personalisation: is the social worker role being eroded? *Community Care Magazine* [online]. Available at: http://www.communitycare.co.uk/Articles/2009/04/01/111172/personalisation-is-the-social-worker-role-being-eroded.htm (accessed June 2010).

Section 10: Personal development and learning

Keeping up-to-date with changes in practice and participating in life-long learning, personal and professional development for one's self and colleagues through supervision, appraisal and reflective practice.

With any helping profession, supervision and reflection are core elements of practice and help to maintain competence and professional development (Clouder, 2000; Payne, 2002). Within mental health this is particularly the case as workers may be dealing with high levels of distress and need to make sure they have the opportunity to analyse their actions and decisions in often difficult circumstances.

> *'...it is necessary to find ways of thoughtful practice a proactive, creative and forward looking activity that allows constant comparisons to be made between actual practice and what is known about best practice'* (Wilshaw & Bohannoh, 2003, p34).

The values that underpin mental health work have shifted from professional values to service user values, which mean that workers need to make sure they are operating according to the individual's preferences and beliefs. This is an activity that can at times be in conflict with the worker's personal beliefs, and as a result, continued reflection is needed. Personalisation reinforces this position, and requires workers and services to respond to individual needs and strengths in a way that is consistent with the person's understanding and experience, with the aim of promoting choice and control and individual rights.

Aims

The use of supervision, appraisal and reflection within mental health support is an activity that can improve practice and hence the experience of service users and carers, and as such, should be a core competence for all those involved. The aim of this final section is to provide an overview of what may be helpful and also signpost individuals to some of the key resources that are available to support reflective practice in personalised mental health support.

- To link professional development and reflective practice with a personalised approach.

Overview

Professional development is more than just accessing training. It involves the individual taking personal responsibility for their learning needs and using a variety of approaches to analyse and reflect on decisions and actions.

Seven areas of competence are included within this shared capability, these are:

Competence 1:	Access to education and training based on the best available evidence.
Competence 2:	A personal/professional development plan that takes account of their hopes and aspirations that is reviewed annually.
Competence 3:	To understand the responsibilities of the service in supporting them in meeting the goals set in the development plan.
Competence 4:	To understand their personal responsibility to achieve the goals set in their development plan.
Competence 5:	The ability to set personal/professional goals that are realistic and achievable.
Competence 6:	To recognise the importance of supervision and reflective practice and integrate both into everyday practice.
Competence 7:	To be proactive in seeking opportunities for personal supervision, personal development and learning.

It is useful for all those involved in delivering support, whether they are workers, service users, or carers to keep themselves up-to-date with developments in the field, and in the case of personalisation, which is a new approach, this is particularly the case. There are many opportunities, both formal and informal, that can be accessed to increase knowledge and experience, and this is necessary in order to maintain competence.

The social approach to disability and mental health issues is an important approach in understanding personalisation and its opportunities, and individuals will benefit from a thorough understanding of this. This is discussed in depth in section 3 of this workbook, however, additional resources are available in the form of an e-learning programme for social workers which has been developed by SCIE, which includes a module on the social approach and how this influences best practice in personalisation. This can be found online at www.scie.org.uk/publications/elearning/person/index.asp

Competence 1

Access to education and training based on the best available evidence.

Personalisation is a relatively new approach, and as such, the evidence base remains limited and far from objective. The involvement and inclusion of people with mental health difficulties is an area that has had some research attention, but as discussed in section 8 this has a definite bias and only includes what is of interest to particular researchers. The best available evidence is often what is the best match for the individual's wants and needs, and to find out what works it may be that options need to be tested out in that person's case. This can make accessing relevant training and education complex, and individuals will need to be aware of their own learning needs and interests in order to fulfil this area of competence. As the Essential Shared Capabilities state (DH, 2004) there is a need for individuals:

> *'...to take an active role in their own personal and professional development. In the same way that service users should be viewed as active partners in their care, not passive recipients, practitioners should be active participants in their own development.'* (p.18)

Within most professional codes of practice there is a requirement for development and learning, however, how this is applied and what is considered relevant is a matter for the individual and their employer or particular situation. Introductions to personalisation and recovery modules are provided in many organisations and this provides a foundation for individuals who are involved in the delivery of personalised mental health support.

Reflection point

What are the areas of your knowledge of personalised mental health that would benefit from further education or training?

One of the key ways to keep up-to-date is to access some of the trade magazines and journals for social care, as well as regularly accessing the internet pages from mental health organisations. These provide news and updates on recent developments as well as details of experiences in the field. The following is a list of some of these resources. It should be noted that this is not comprehensive and individuals will need to explore what is available to meet their individual learning and development needs.

It should be remembered that while national resources are useful sources of information there is also a need for individuals to identify what is available to them locally via their local training departments and other community opportunities.

Selected resources

Mental Health Today magazine
www.pavpub.com/pavpub/magazines/mht/

Community Care magazine:
www.communitycare.co.uk

National Mental Health Development Unit (NMHDU)
www.nmhdu.org.uk

NMHDU Paths to Personalisation
www.pathstopersonalisation.org.uk

Social Care Institute for Excellence (SCIE)
www.scie.org.uk

Social Perspectives Network
www.spn.org.uk

Department of Health Care Networks: Personalisation network
http://www.dhcarenetworks.org.uk/personalisation/index.cfm

Department of Health Personalisation Section
www.dh.gov.uk/en/SocialCare/Socialcarereform/Personalisation/index.htm

Putting People First
www.puttingpeoplefirst.org.uk/

Competence 2

A personal/professional development plan that takes account of their hopes and aspirations that is reviewed annually.

Development plans have been introduced into most professions over the last decade, and organisations are often required to support staff to develop these plans as part of their employment. For service users, carers or other informal supporters this approach is also beneficial as it clarifies the personal and professional needs and encourages a culture of learning throughout all activities. Development plans can take a variety of forms, however, the common themes should include – training needs, supervision requirements, the aspirations of the individual and role related learning. Competence-based learning, such as that set out throughout this workbook, provides a clear link between learning and the area of work or support. In the case of mental health work, power and engagement issues should also be considered as these can directly contribute to risk enablement processes which increase the choice and control for individuals who access support.

In social care terms there are requirements of both the worker and the employer within the social care code of practice in relation to learning and development, and these apply to the personalisation approach. The General Social Care Council (GSCC) is the registration authority for social work and social care, and the code states:

> *'As a social care worker, you must be accountable for the quality of your work and take responsibility for maintaining and improving your knowledge and skills.'*
> (GSCC, 2002, p17)

> *'As a social care employer, you must provide training and development opportunities to enable social care workers to strengthen and develop their skills and knowledge.'*
> (GSCC, 2002, p29)

However, it must be remembered that delivering personalised support for mental health issues is part of both health and social care, and as such, everyone involved needs to take responsibility for ensuring that individuals have development plans which are relevant to their roles and improve their competence. A lot of mental health care is delivered by integrated health and social care services managed through the NHS and the personalised approach needs to be embedded in integrated services (Duffy, 2010).

Reflection points

- What are your hopes and aspirations for the support you provide or receive?
- What are your personal and professional goals – both short-term (in the next 6–12 months) and longer-term (in the next five years)?
- How does your development plan help to meet these goals?

As a final issue, all training and development issues should include equality and diversity considerations and cultural competency training, and the range of issues highlighted in sections 3 and 4 of this workbook. In particular, the implications of the Equality Bill for training and professional development need to be explored. Staff must be able to provide a service to all citizens regardless of race, age, gender, disability, sexual orientation, age and faith and the ability to do so is a performance, management and personal development issue that should be embedded within all development planning processes.

Competence 3

To understand the responsibilities of the service in supporting them in meeting the goals set in the development plan.

As noted in competence 2, there is a responsibility on the employer to support workers in their professional development. These requirements will vary according to role and profession, and in some disciplines, such as social care (GSCC, 2002). This is an explicit responsibility within the codes of practice.

Workforce development is an area that has been considered within mental health and central policy reinforces this, with New Horizons (DH, 2009) making specific reference to the need for development in recognition that a skilled workforce is an essential requirement for improving the experience and outcomes for those who access the service.

> *'Within mental health, it is vital that staff be well led, supported and supervised, and have access to continuing professional development locally.'* (DH, 2009, p80)

Putting People First, the concordat that sets out the strategy for personalisation, also recognised that the workforce would need development and support to implement the changes in support delivery, with the following objective:

> *'Local workforce development strategies focused on raising skill levels ... across all sectors. Strategies to be co-produced, co-developed and co-evaluated with the private and voluntary sectors.'* (HM Government, 2007, p4)

In addition to the professional development of workers, there is also an emphasis on supporting and developing user-led organisations. The focus here is on taking a partnership approach to learning, with service users and carers developing and delivering training and being able to access development opportunities, and organisations enabling access to training for local user-led organisations (HM Government, 2009).

The personalisation agenda sets out a vision that there should be a user-led organisation (ULO) in each area by 2010 (Cabinet Office, 2005; HM Government 2009; SCIE, 2009), and traditional providers need to support and engage with these organisations with the aim of increasing user control and listening to the voice of those who access services.

The definition of a ULO is an organisation that is run by, and controlled by, people who use support services. The overall aims of ULOs are to promote independent living and some of their activities include:

- information and advice
- advocacy and peer support
- support in using direct payments and/or individual budgets
- support to recruit and employ personal assistants
- assistance with self-assessment
- disability equality training
- support implementation of the disability equality duty.

The Department of Health has set criteria that organisations must meet to be classed as a ULO, and this includes a set of values centred on the social model of disability and organisational requirements including accountability to those who use the services and inclusion of all service user groups (DH, 2007; DH, 2009). There is evidence that shows that the involvement of ULOs in service delivery and evaluation has a range of benefits (Swain *et al*, 2004; HM Government, 2009; SCIE, 2009; DH, 2010) including more flexible and user-centred services, increased employment opportunities and greater community involvement.

In mental health there have been many barriers to accessing direct payments (Newbigging & Lowe, 2005; Spandler & Vick, 2005) and this is mirrored in the uptake of personal budgets and the slow progression towards a personalised approach for this group. ULOs have taken on the support and brokerage role in many areas, however, it seems that there has been a further barrier and many individuals have not been made aware of the support they could access via their local ULO (Davidson & Luckhurst, 2002; Spandler & Vick, 2005).

Reflection points

- Is there a user-led organisation in your area?
- What services are provided by your ULO?
- What impact does this have on involvement and service provision?
- How do you/could you engage with your local ULO?

Competence 4

To understand their personal responsibility to achieve the goals set in their development plan.

Individual development plans are part of the learning process but they need to be working documents that are worked through and delivered. For this to be the case, plans need to match personal aspirations and be relevant to the individual's role. While the employer or service provider has a responsibility to support the person in their plan, the person themself also needs to take personal responsibility for ensuring they take an active role in their own continued development.

The focus on choice and control within the personalised approach is mirrored here, as individuals need to be able to take control of their learning and reflect on what they need to be able to provide person-centred support. This responsibility includes being able to identify both skills and needs, and set goals that will help the individual in their role of providing mental health support within a personalised context. Ongoing reflection is one way to achieve this aim, and while attending training can be useful, this in itself is not sufficient. The individual needs to be able to apply the learning to their practice and incorporate it into the day-to-day skills.

Activity

Think about the last training or learning event you attended, or the last document you read concerning personalisation and complete the following task.

What was the activity? And what were the key messages?	
What goal did it meet from your development plan?	
What were the objectives of the activity and did it meet these? Specify how and why.	
How will you put this into practice (what difference has it made)?	
What are your future learning needs that were highlighted by the activity?	

Competence 5

The ability to set personal/professional goals that are realistic and achievable.

The SMART planning process that was explored in section 7 of this workbook applies to development goals in the same way as it does for recovery goals, and individuals need to ensure that their plans are specific, realistic and achievable. The changes in the way services are organised and delivered presents a challenge to the large traditional organisations as they have a history and culture that has developed over time, which can be a struggle to change. For those involved in delivering personal support there is a real shift, and service user values and agendas need to be central to the development of staff, volunteers and individuals.

Balancing risk and empowerment can be a challenge to workers and services, and mental health in particular has been an area where the user voice has not been as powerful as it could be within the personalised approach. Safety and risk have been the clinical emphasis, and there is also a range of stigmatising attitudes and presumptions made about individuals, based on worker anxiety and prejudicial views of capacity and ability, which are often less to do with the person's capability than a pervading view that those with mental health issues need protection above all else. This issue has been a barrier to individuals exercising choice and control in their care and support, and as such, is an area that needs to be addressed in the learning and development of service providers and individual workers.

Safeguarding is an area that has recently been reviewed (DH, 2000; DH, 2009) and personalisation presents specific challenges for social care providers. The recent review of *No Secrets* (DH, 2009) identified the need for education, training and guidance for all involved to be able to deliver personalisation in a safeguarding framework:

> *'...it should look at positive risk assessment and monitoring and safeguarding and empowerment all in one. Do not separate them, because each is only part of the picture.'* (DH, 2009, p29)

As a result those within mental health services would benefit from development goals that reflect this balance and respond to the anxiety of services in implementing the approach.

Reflective activity

Write yourself a development goal that would help you to balance safeguarding and choice and control, and ask yourself the following questions. Is your goal achievable in the next 12 months? Is it realistic in your context? Is it specific?

Competence 6

To recognise the importance of supervision and reflective practice and integrate both into everyday practice.

Supervision can mean different things to different people in different contexts, and it is useful to first define what is meant here by the term before considering how it can impact on the implementation and delivery of personalised mental health. From a social care perspective, supervision can be a one-to-one or group activity, and essentially is time set aside for the individual to analyse, reflect and learn about the actions and decisions they have, or intend to make and identify their development needs. It has a number of functions that can be summarised into three categories (Kadushin, 1992; McKenna *et al*, 2008):

- education/learning – learning from experiences by reflecting on activities, encouraging development and identifying learning needs
- management/performance – monitoring activity and setting performance goals
- support – supporting the individual in their role and context.

Within this framework the main purpose of supervision is to influence the ability of the individual to provide effective support to service users (and carers) (Wampold & Holloway, 1997) and research has shown that effective supervision impacts on both the working relationship (Bambling *et al*, 2006) and can contribute to improving individual outcomes and recovery (Blatt *et al*, 1996; Krupnick *et al*, 1996; Wampold, 2001).

Reflection, both personal and professional, is a major component of supervision, and means that the individual critically analyses their practice to inform learning and future practice. This includes considering decisions and actions, as well as the rationale for interventions and the values that they are based upon (Ruth-Sahd, 2003; Taylor, 2006). While a person can reflect individually, with tools such as reflective logs and journals being popular in professional education, supervision is the opportunity for discussion and unpacking the various elements of practice with another person, whose role it is to provide both challenge and support. There are a number of models and tools for reflection that can be used to help in this process, and individuals will need to develop their own preferred styles. Challenging personal views and prejudices should form part of this process, and form the foundation for all antidiscriminatory training and practice supervision.

The impact that supervision and reflective practice has on both the working relationship and positive user outcomes is well documented and these can be applied across the personalisation approach. A study carried out by Ruth-Sahd in 2003, which evaluated a range of studies on the importance of reflective practice highlighted the following benefits documented within the literature for workers:

- development of knowledge and skills
- integration of theoretical concepts to practice
- increased learning from experience
- improvement in practice by enabling greater self-awareness
- enhanced critical thinking and the ability to make judgements in complex and uncertain situations
- acceptance of professional responsibility and continuous professional growth
- improved self-worth through learning.

In terms of the impact on service user and carer experience, the improvement that can be achieved through reflective practice has a direct impact on those who access the service. As such, it can be suggested that reflective practice and the effective use of supervision have much to contribute to the improvement in individual outcomes.

Activity

Choose an intervention you have been involved in that is part of a personalised approach – this could be an assessment, developing a support plan, providing a direct payment or individual budget or another action or decision you have made. Follow the stages of the model listed below (Gibbs, 1988) for the issue you have identified – complete the exercise alone and then again with your supervisor or a friend or colleague, compare your reflections from each situation and identify what was useful and what you have learnt from the two experiences.

- **Stage 1:** Description of the event – Describe the event in detail. Where were you? Who else was there? Why were you there? What were you doing? What were other people doing? What was the context of the event? What happened? What was your part in this? What parts did the other people play? What was the result?
- **Stage 2**: Feelings and thoughts (self-awareness) – How were you feeling when the event started? What were you thinking about at the time? How did it make you feel? How did you feel about the outcome of the event? What do you think about it now?
- **Stage 3:** Evaluation – Evaluate or make a judgement about what happened. Consider what was good about the experience and what was bad about the experience or what did or didn't go so well.
- **Stage 4:** Analysis – What went well? What did you do well? What went wrong or did not turn out how it should have done? In what way did you or others contribute to this?
- **Stage 5**: Conclusion (synthesis) – How did you contribute to the outcome of the event. You should ask yourself what you could have done differently.
- **Stage 6:** Action plan – In a similar situation would you act differently or would you be likely to do the same?

Competence 7

To be proactive in seeking opportunities for personal supervision, personal development and learning.

Identifying opportunities to meet personal and professional development, learning and supervision needs is the responsibility of the individual, and while the organisation must support development, the person themself needs to take responsibility and control their own learning processes.

There are many activities, events and resources available to support development of competence and knowledge in regard to personalisation, and these will continue to be developed as the approach is put into place. Internet resources, journals, trade magazines, local and national organisations and networks have been established and these will assist in the updating of individuals on current progress and initiatives. These should be discussed in supervision or peer learning activities to help the individual to apply this learning to practice.

Activity

Identify at least two internet sites that can be used to develop knowledge and skills in personalisation for mental health.

- What are the resources?

- What information and learning can be gained from these resources?

- How will this information influence your activities and role?

Formal training courses are often seen as the means by which learning is achieved, however, this is just one part of the picture and other methods such as discussion, reading, visiting other projects, shadowing workers and online activities also need to be included in the activities of the individual. Examples of good practice are being collected by the Department of Health and SCIE (among others) and these can be used to inform local activities and projects, and all those involved in implementing personalisation need to remain aware of the experience of others and what lessons can be learnt from these experiences.

Summary

This capability has considered the area of continuing professional development and how training, resources and supervision can be used to inform activities and implement personalisation within mental health settings. The requirements of this capability are:

'Keeping up-to-date with changes in practice and participating in life-long learning, personal and professional development for one's self and colleagues through supervision, appraisal and reflective practice.'

There is a range of means by which this can be achieved and individuals need to take personal responsibility for their development needs. Different methods and formats can be accessed to support this area and regardless of role – whether service user, carer or worker, there is a wealth of sources that can be accessed. The use of groups and networks, as well as organisations such as SCIE and NMHDU, are means by which up-to-date information can be accessed, and while there are limitations due to the newness of the approach, these will continue to develop as research, experience and examples of good practice are tested out and evaluated.

Summary exercise

Write a short summary of what this capability means to you in your context/practice, and then answer the following three questions.

- What have you learnt by completing this section?

- How have you now reached competence in this area?

- What do you need to do to maintain your competence?

References

Bambling M, King R, Raue P, Schweitzer R & Lambert W (2006) Clinical supervision: its influence on client-rated working alliance and client symptom reduction in the brief treatment of major depression. *Psychotherapy Research* **16** 317–331.

Blatt SJ, Zuroff DC, Quinlan DM & Pilkonis PA (1996) Interpersonal factors in brief treatment of depression: further analysis of the National Institute of Mental Health treatment of depression collaborative research program. *Journal of Consulting and Clinical Psychology* **64** 162–171.

Cabinet Office (2005) *Improving the Life Chances of Disabled People*. London: TSO.

Clouder L (2000) Reflective practice in physiotherapy. *Studies in Higher Education* **25** (2) 211–223.

Davidson D & Luckhurst L (2002) *Making Choices, Taking Control: Direct payments and mental health service users/survivors*. York: Joseph Rowntree Foundation.

Department of Health (2000) *No Secrets: Guidance on developing and implementing multi-agency policies and procedures to protect vulnerable adults from abuse*. London: DH.

Department of Health (2004) *The 10 Shared Capabilities: A framework for the whole of the mental health workforce*. London: TSO.

Department of Health (2007) *User-led Organisations Project: Policy*. London: DH.

Department of Health (2009) *Safeguarding Adults: Report on the consultation on the review of No Secrets*. London: DH.

Department of Health (2010) *Sharing the Learning: User-led organisations action and learning sites* 2008–2010. London: DH.

Duffy S (2010) *Personalisation in Mental Health*. Sheffield: Centre for Welfare Reform/ Yorkshire & Humberside Improvement Partnership, Care Pathways & Packages Project & ADASS.

General Social Care Council (GSCC) (2002) *Codes of Practice for Social Care Workers and Employers*. London: GSCC.

Gibbs G (1988) *Learning by Doing: A guide to teaching and learning methods*. Oxford: Further Education Unit.

HM Government (2007) *Putting People First: A shared vision and commitment to the transformation of adult social care*. London: TSO.

HM Government (2009) *Putting People First: Working together with user-led organisations*. London: TSO.

Kadushin A (1992) *Supervision in Social Work* (3rd ed). New York: Columbia University Press.

Krupnick JL, Simmens S, Moyer J, Elkin I, Watkins JT & Pilkonis PA (1996) The role of the therapeutic alliance in psychotherapy and pharmacotherapy outcome: findings in the National Institute of Mental Health treatment of depression collaborative research program. *Journal of Consulting and Clinical Psychology* **64** 532–539.

McKenna B, Thom K, Howard F & Williams V (2008) *Professional Supervision for Mental Health and Addiction Nurses: A review of current approaches to professional supervision internationally and in the New Zealand mental health and addiction sector*. Auckland: National Centre of Mental Health Research, Information and Workforce Development.

Newbigging K & Lowe J (2005) *Direct Payments and Mental Health: New directions*. Brighton: Pavilion Publishing.

Payne M (2002) Social work theories and reflective practice. In: L Dominelli, M Payne & R Adams (Eds) *Social Work: Themes, issues and critical debates*. (2nd ed). Basingstoke: Palgrave/Open University.

Ruth-Sahd LA (2003) Reflective practice: a critical analysis of data-based studies and implications for nursing practice. *Journal of Nursing Education* **42** (11) 488–497.

SCIE (2009) *At A Glance 15: Personalisation briefing – Implications for user-led organisations* [online]. London: SCIE. Available at: http://www.scie.org.uk/publications/ataglance/ataglance15.pdf (accessed June 2010).

Spandler H & Vick N (2005) Enabling Access to Direct Payments: an exploration of care co-ordinators decision-making practices. *Journal of Mental Health* **14** (2) 145–155.

Swain J, French S, Barnes C & Thomas C (Eds) (2004) *Disabling Barriers, Enabling environments*. London: SAGE.

Taylor C (2006) Narrating significant experience: reflective accounts and the production of (self) knowledge. *British Journal of Social Work* **36** (2) 189–206.

Wampold BE (2001) *The Great Psychotherapy Debate: Models, methods, and findings*. Mahway, NJ: Lawrence Erlbaum Associates.

Wampold BE & Holloway EL (1997) Methodology, design, and evaluation in psychotherapy supervision research. In: CE Watkins Jr (Ed) *Handbook of Psychotherapy Supervision* (pp11–27). Hoboken, NJ: John Wiley & Sons.

Wilshaw G & Bohannoh N (2003) Reflective practice and team teaching in mental health care. *Nursing Standard* **17** (50) 33–37.